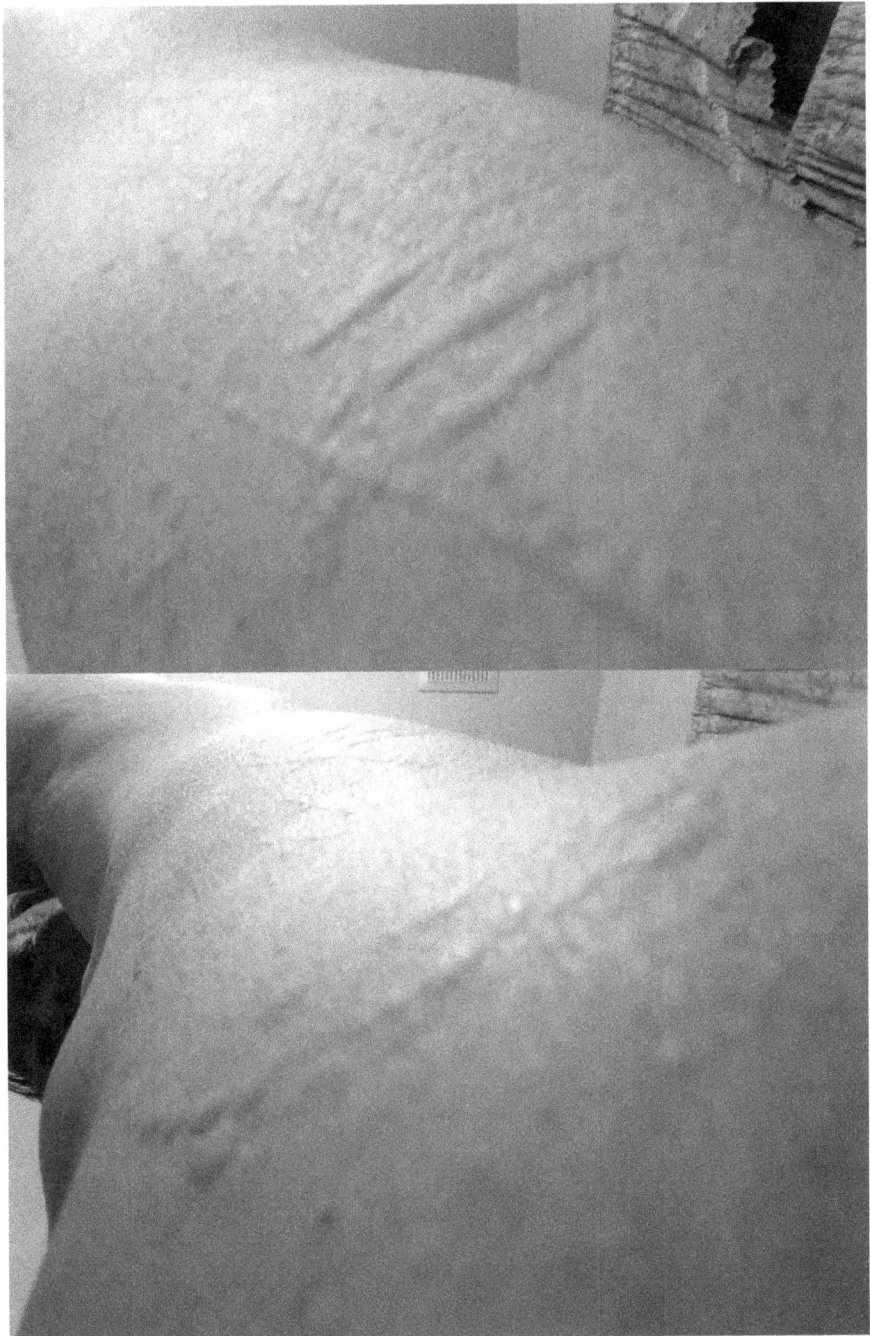

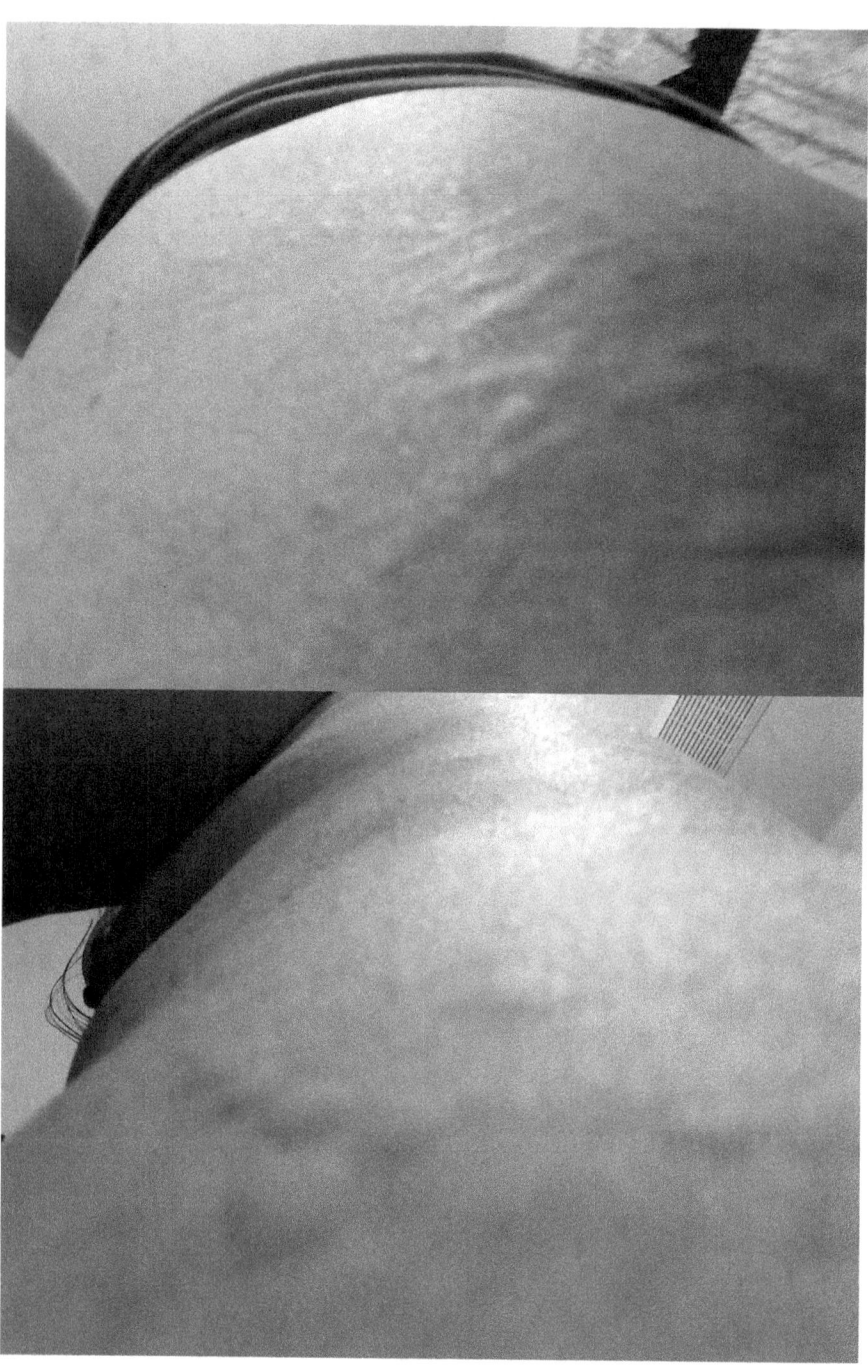

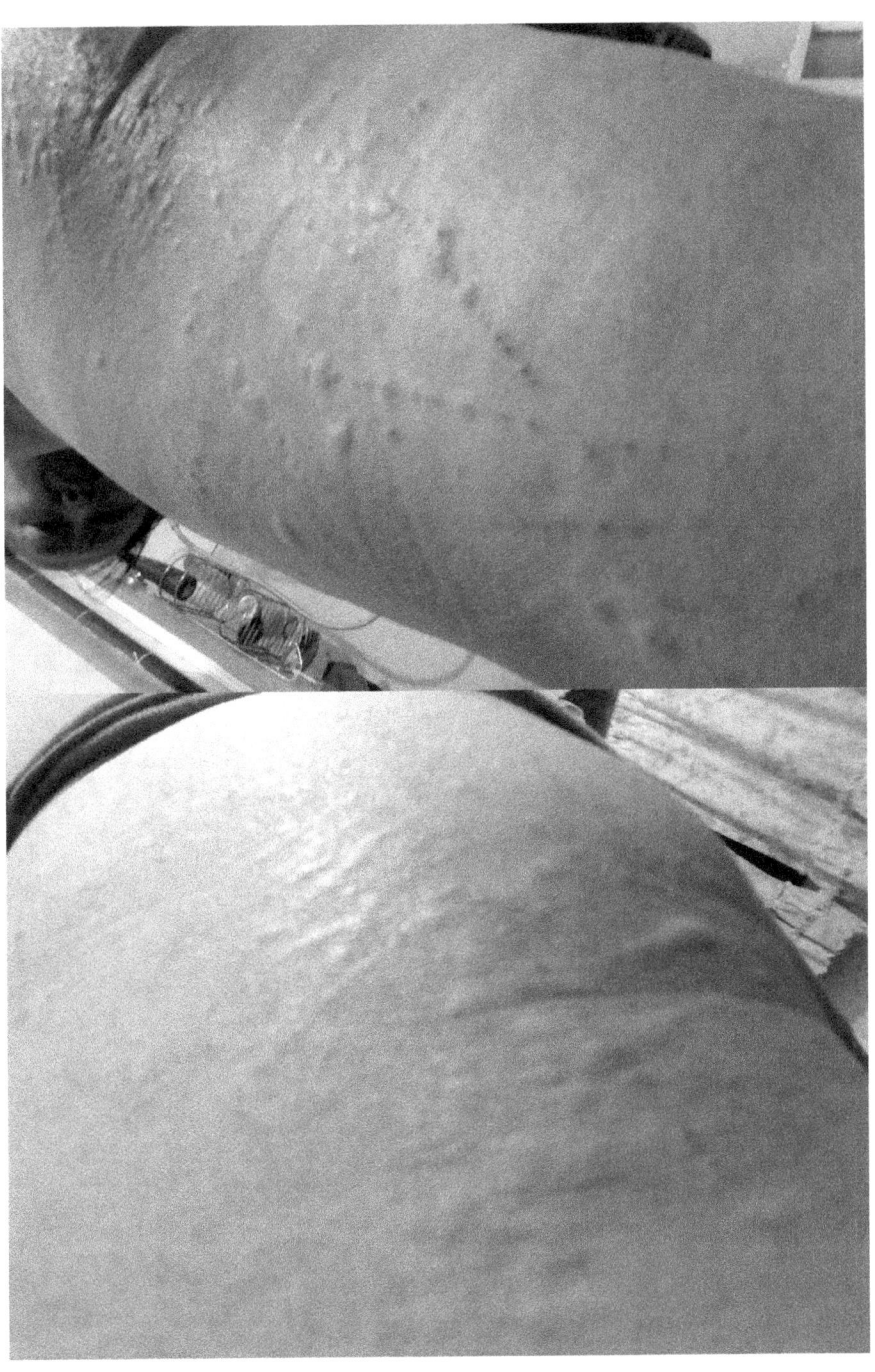

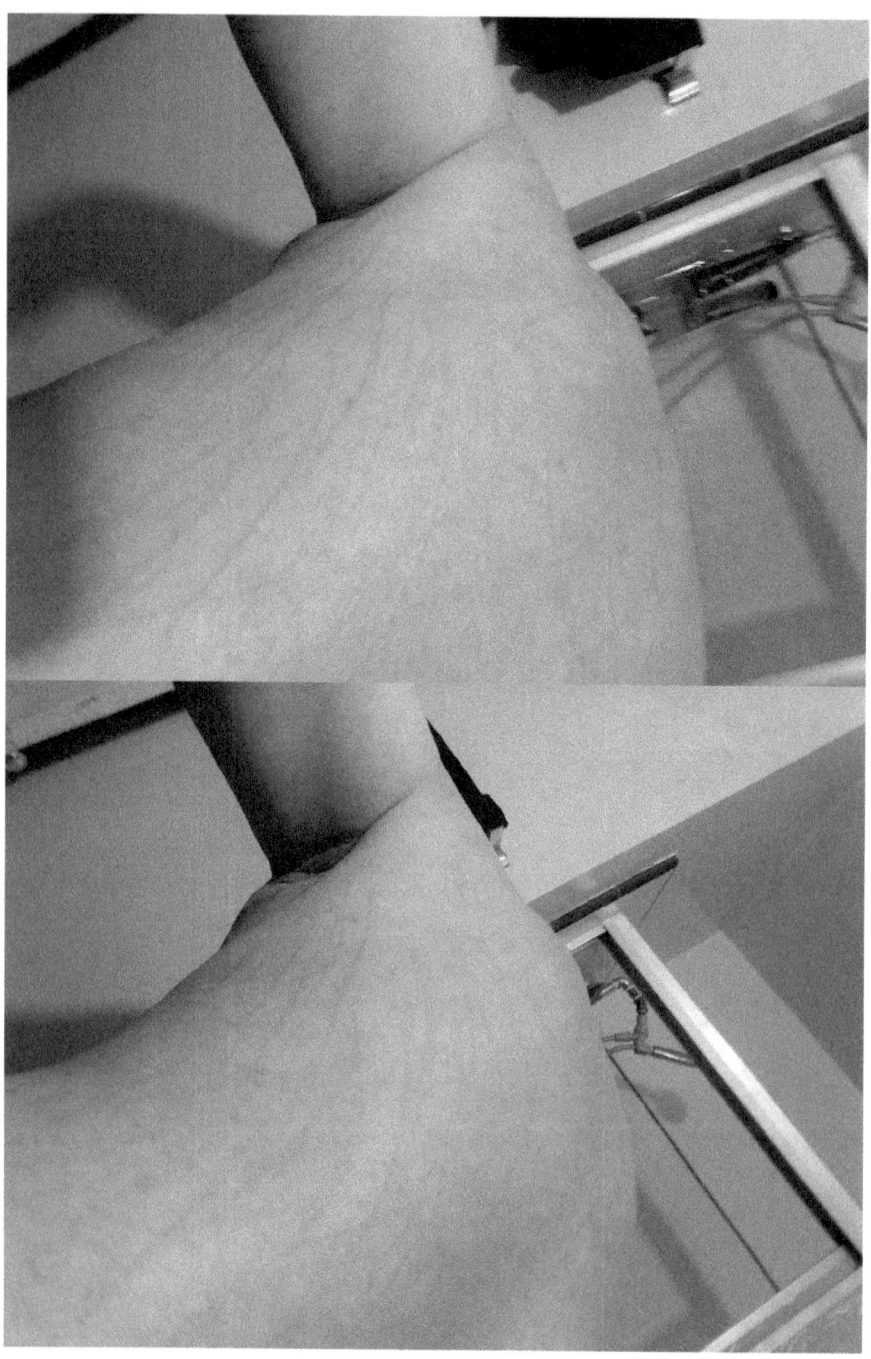

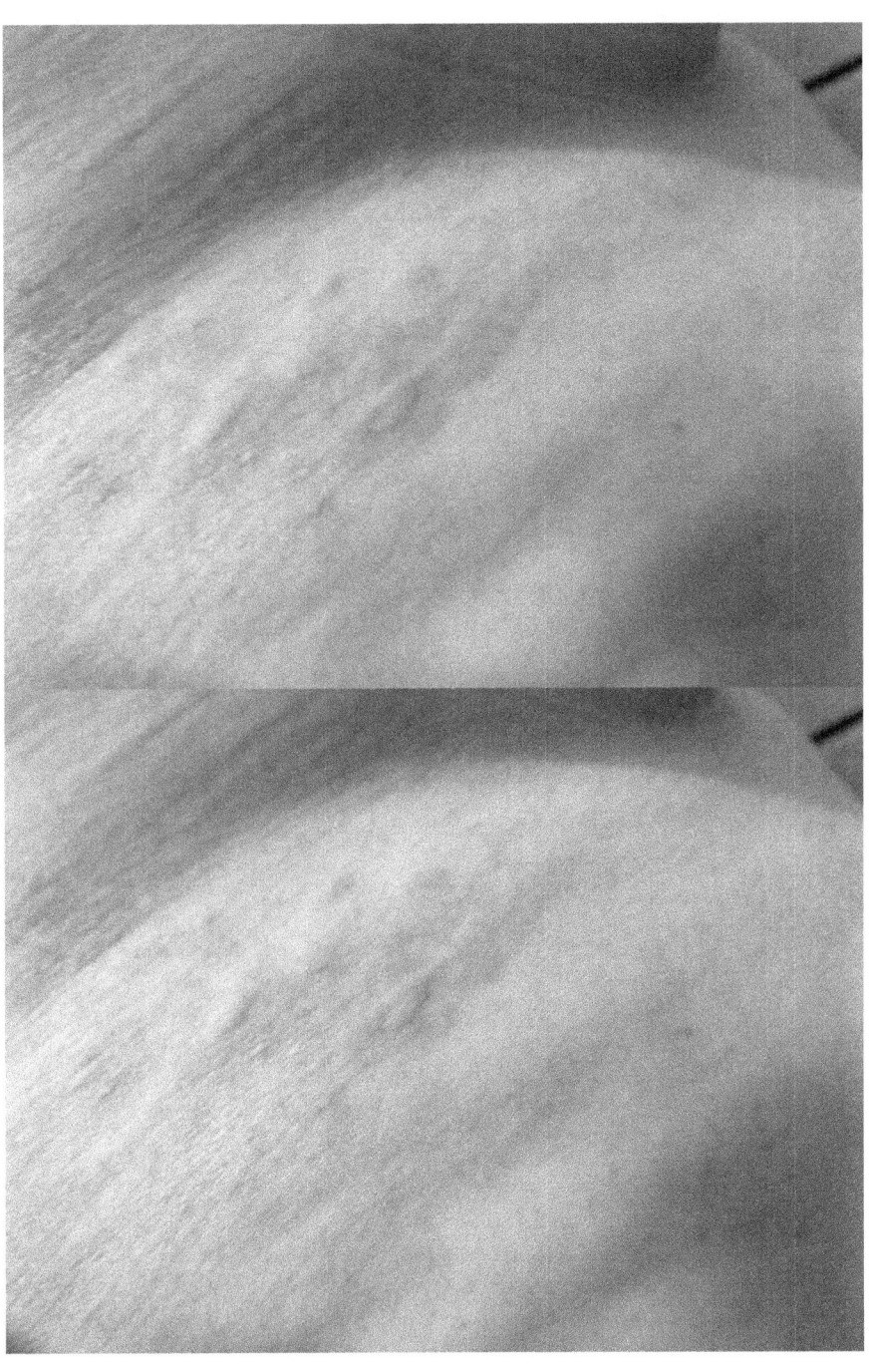

There are several types of hives accompanied by itching:

1. **welts**
2. **scratches**
3. **bumps**

Hives can be caused by many factors, most commonly due to food allergies, such as reaction to fish, mercury, and may indicate early stages of kidney and/or liver disease. Various tests can be administered to determine the causes. Antihistamines and topical ointments are often prescribed by doctors to treat the symptoms, but usually are not effective in mediating the causes or severity of symptoms that tend to go away within a day if the allergen is not continued. Check with your doctor if you get any of these symptoms and patterns.

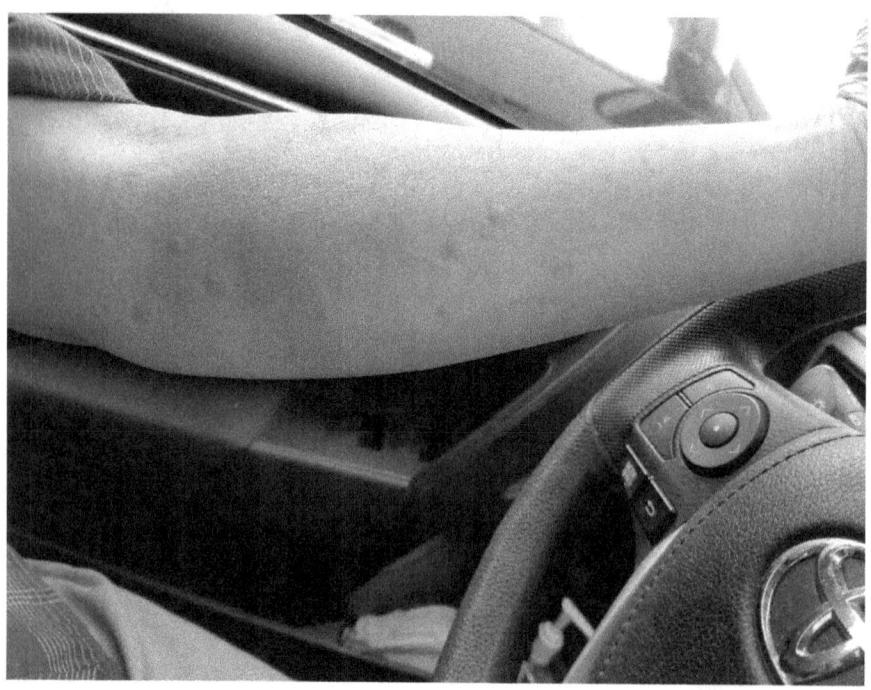

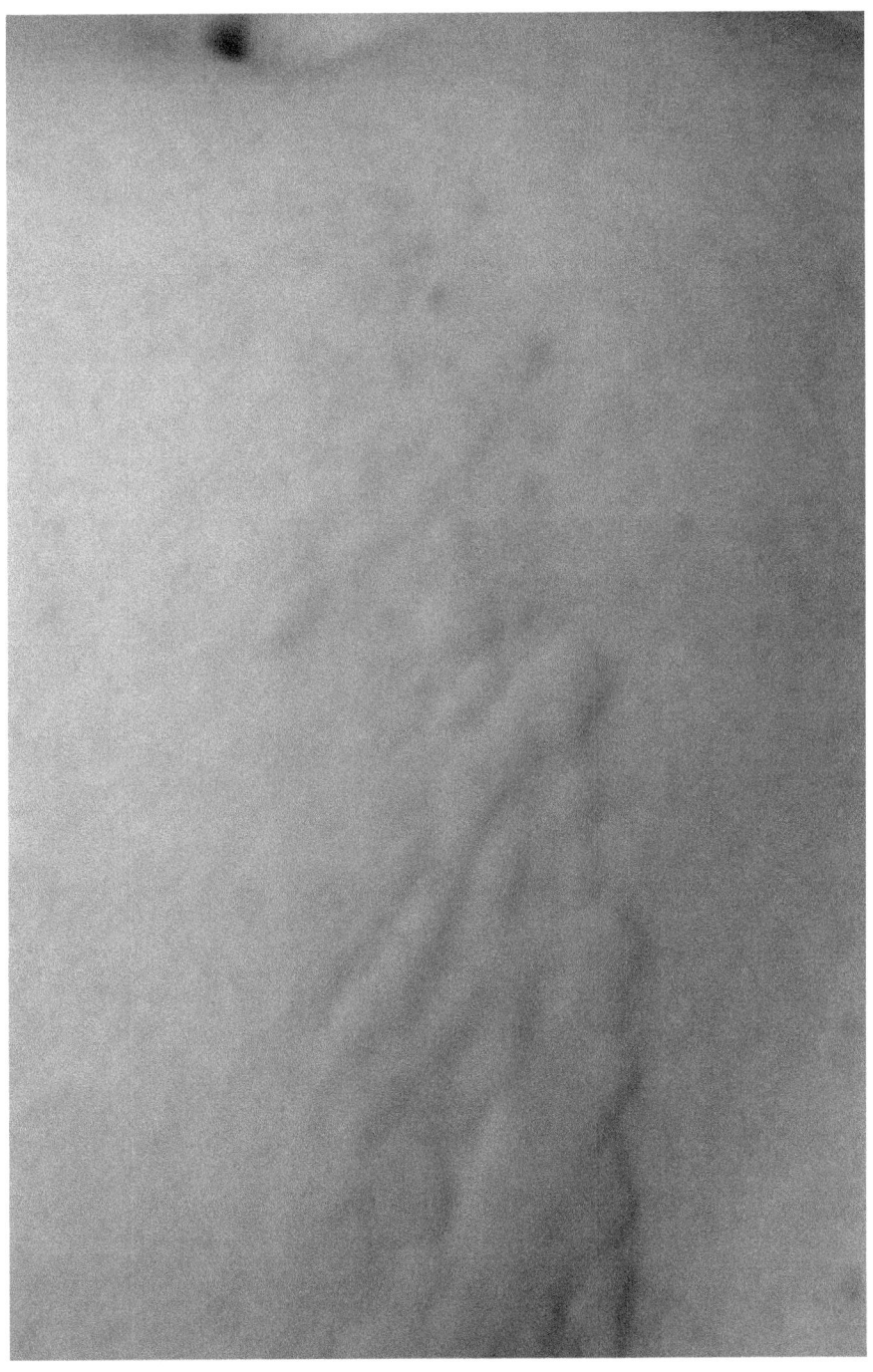

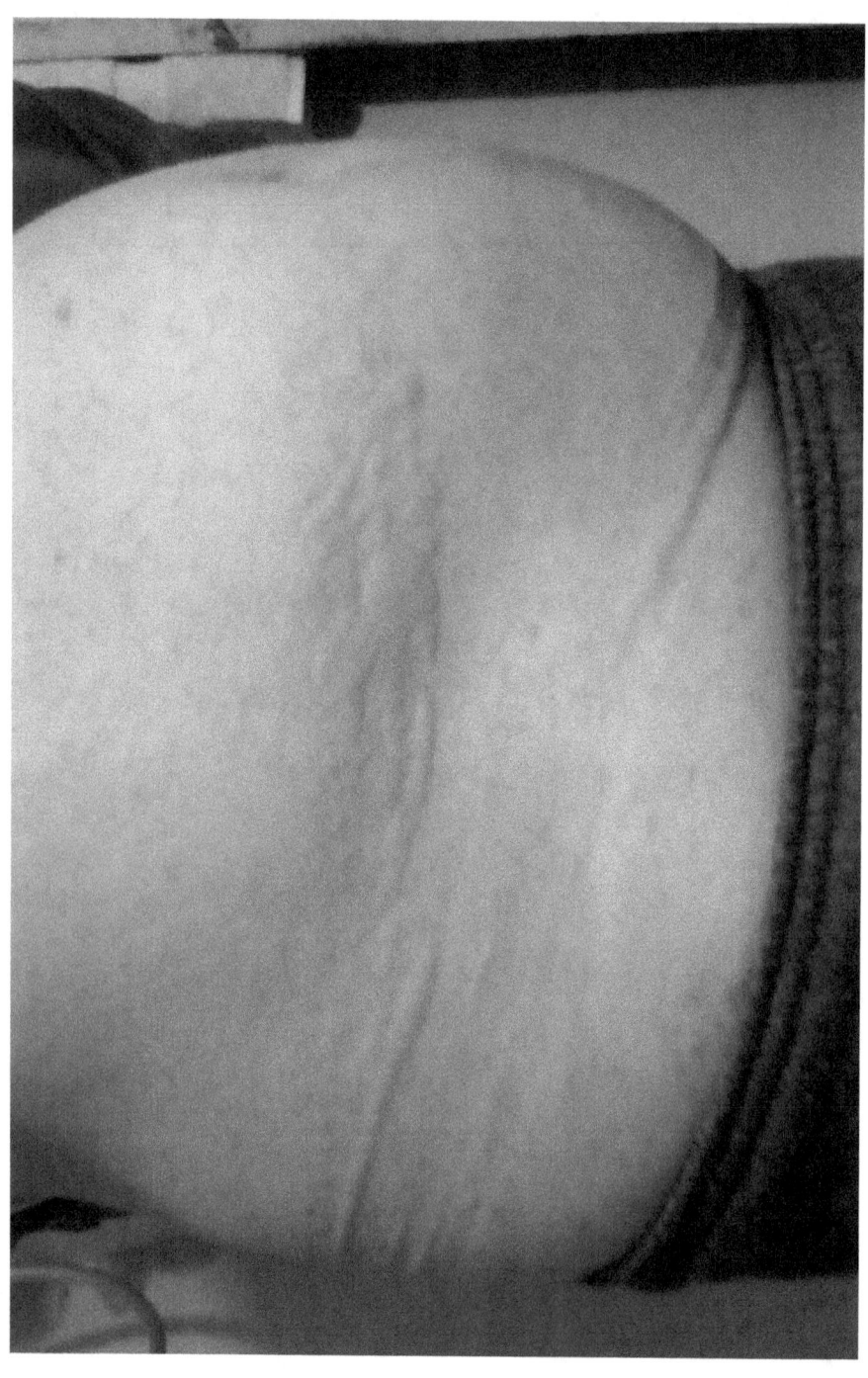

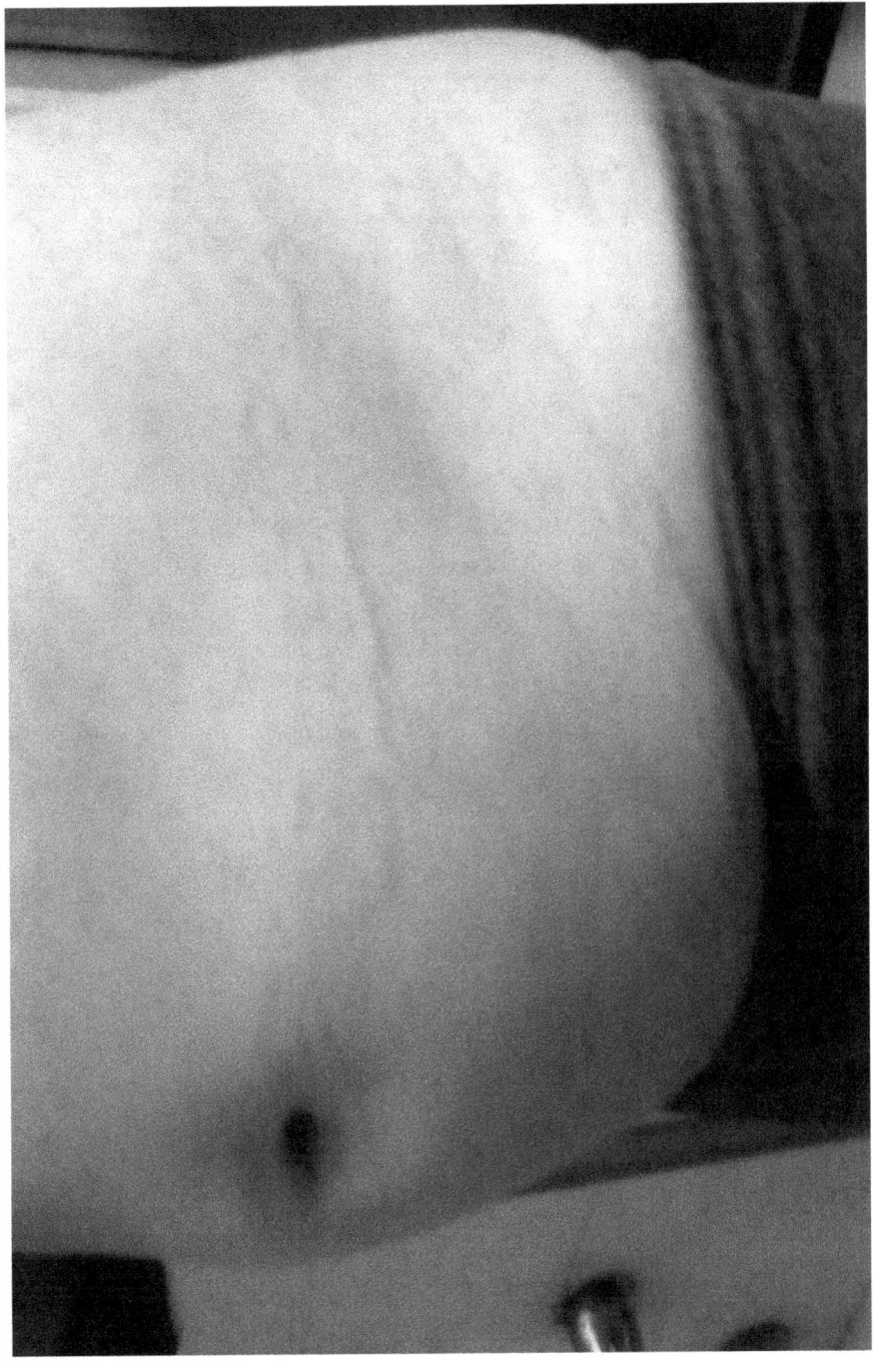

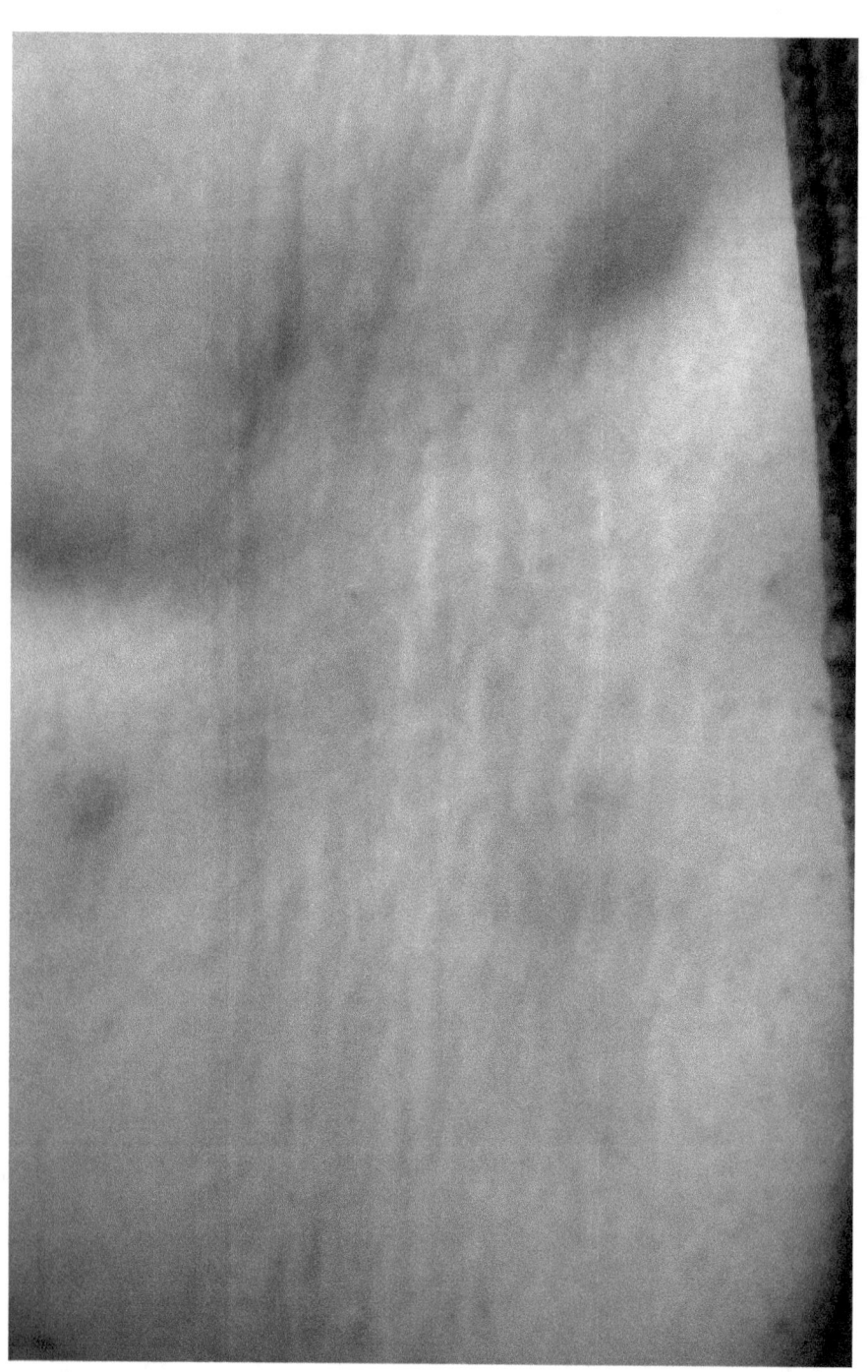

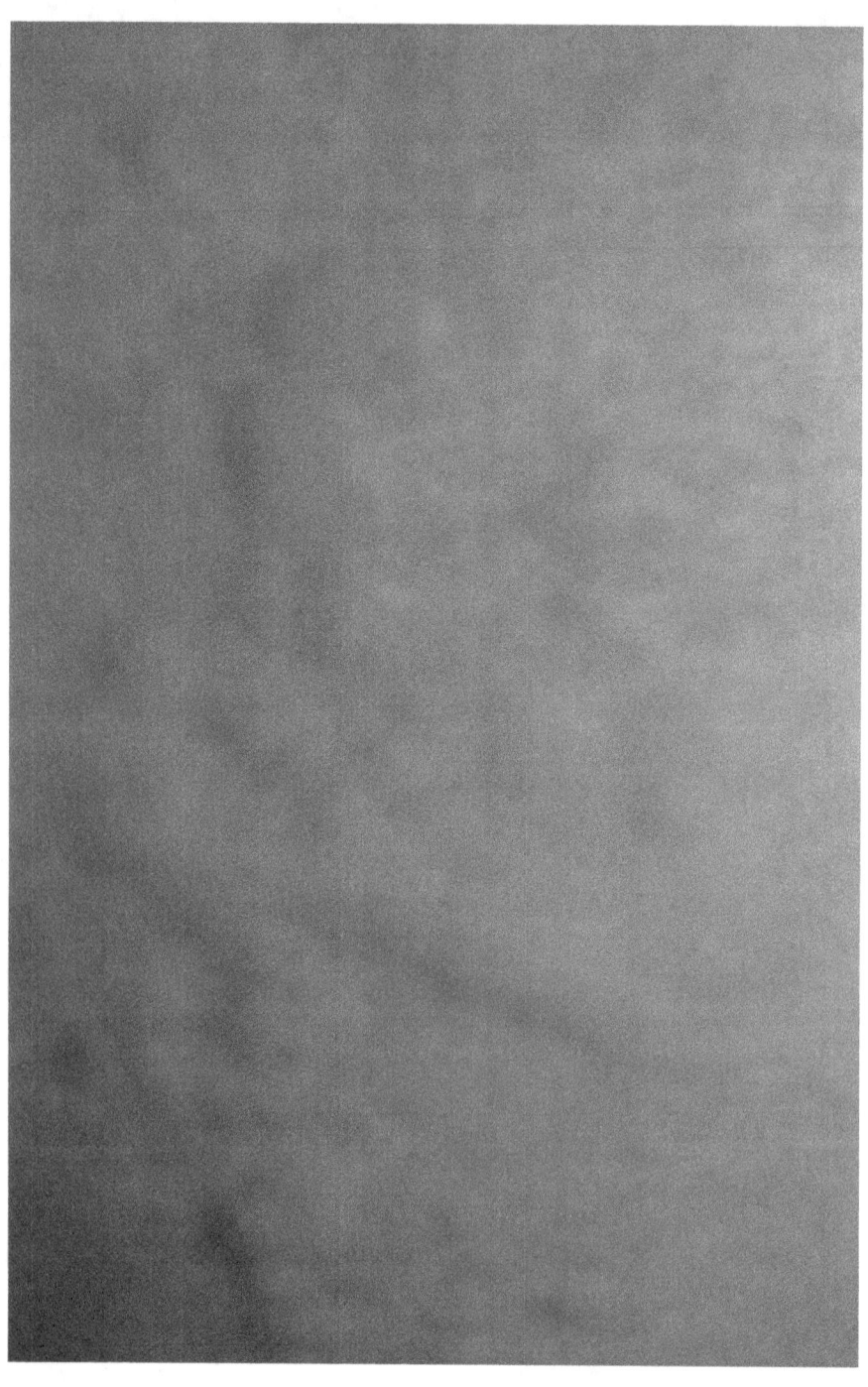

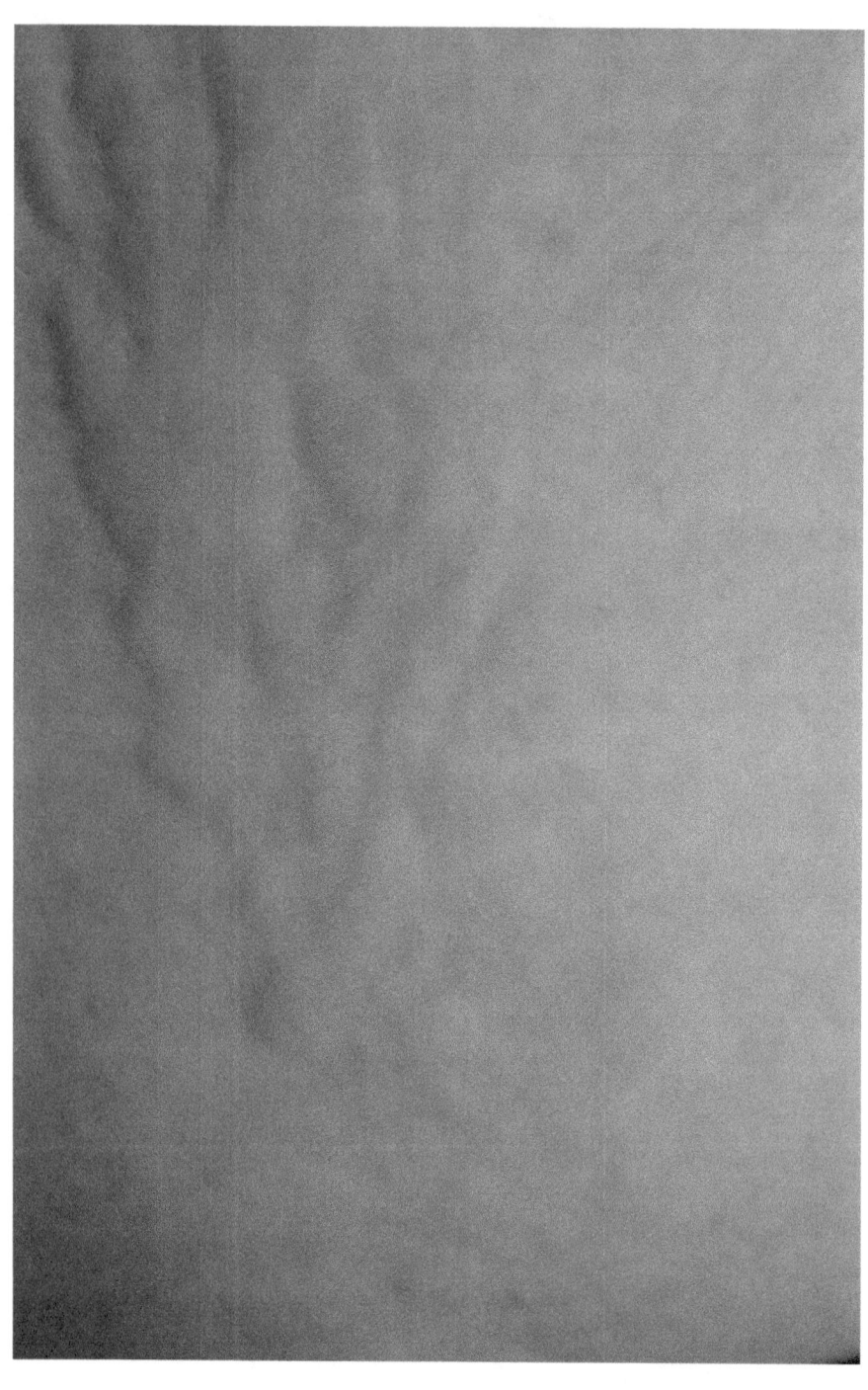

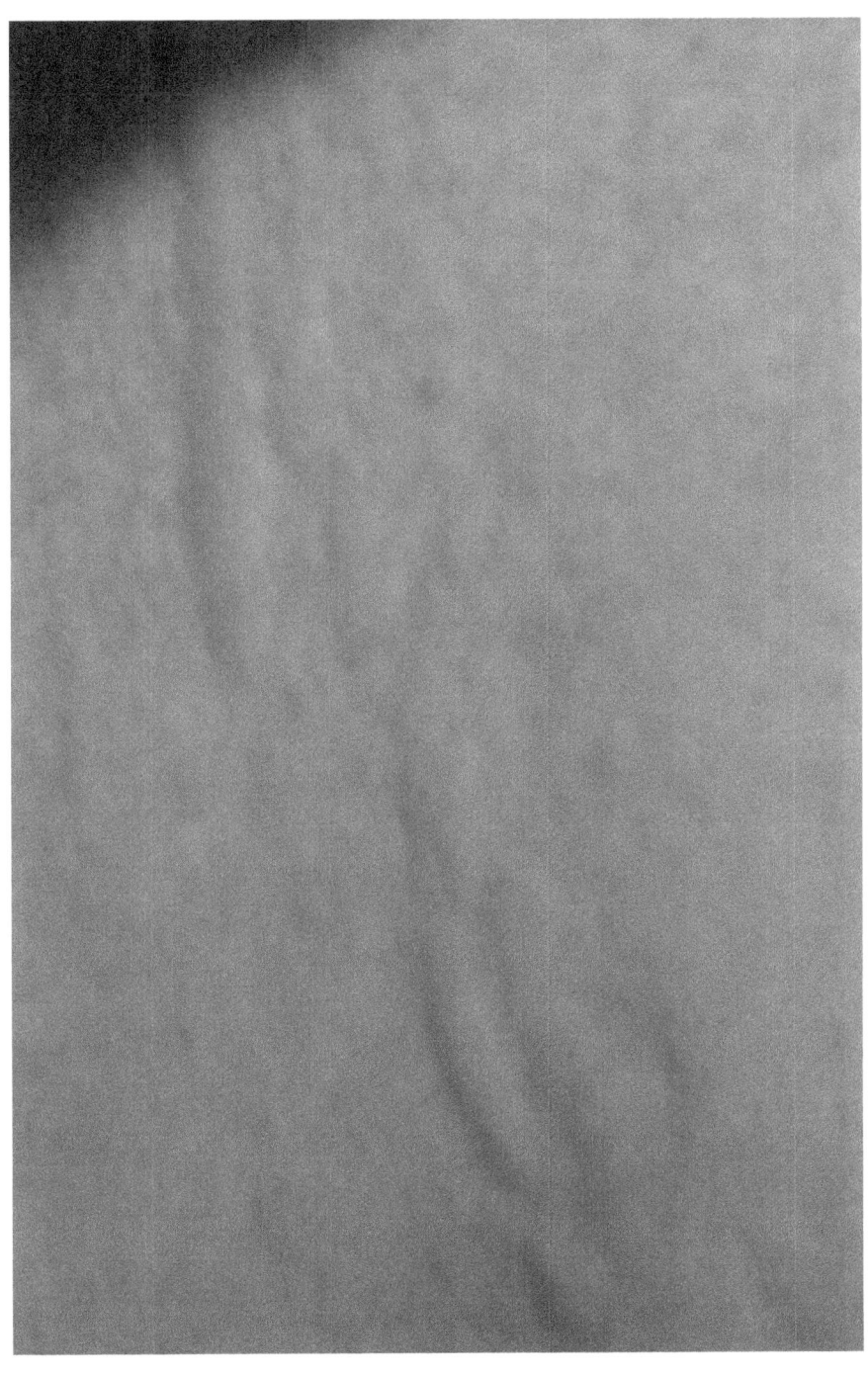

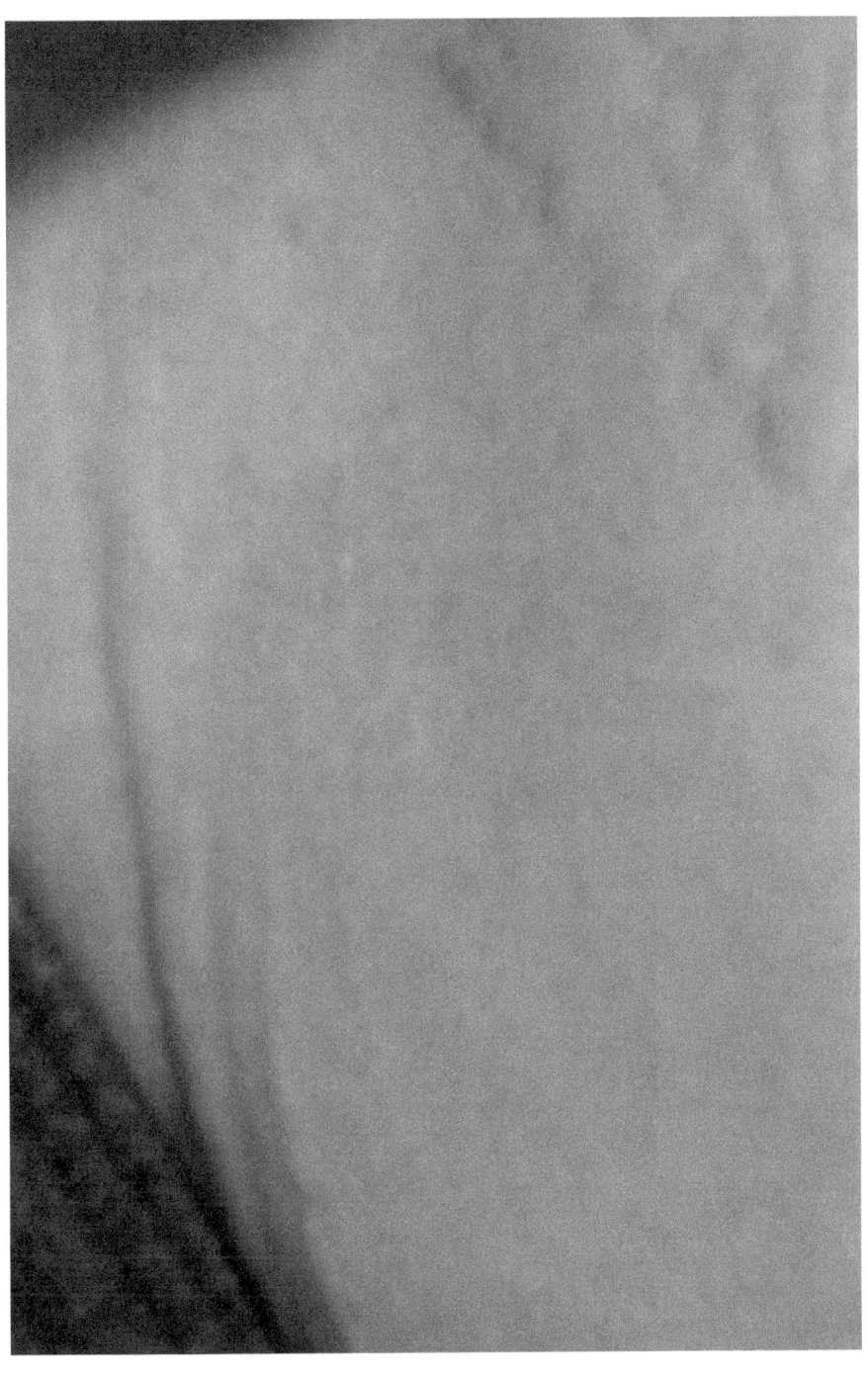

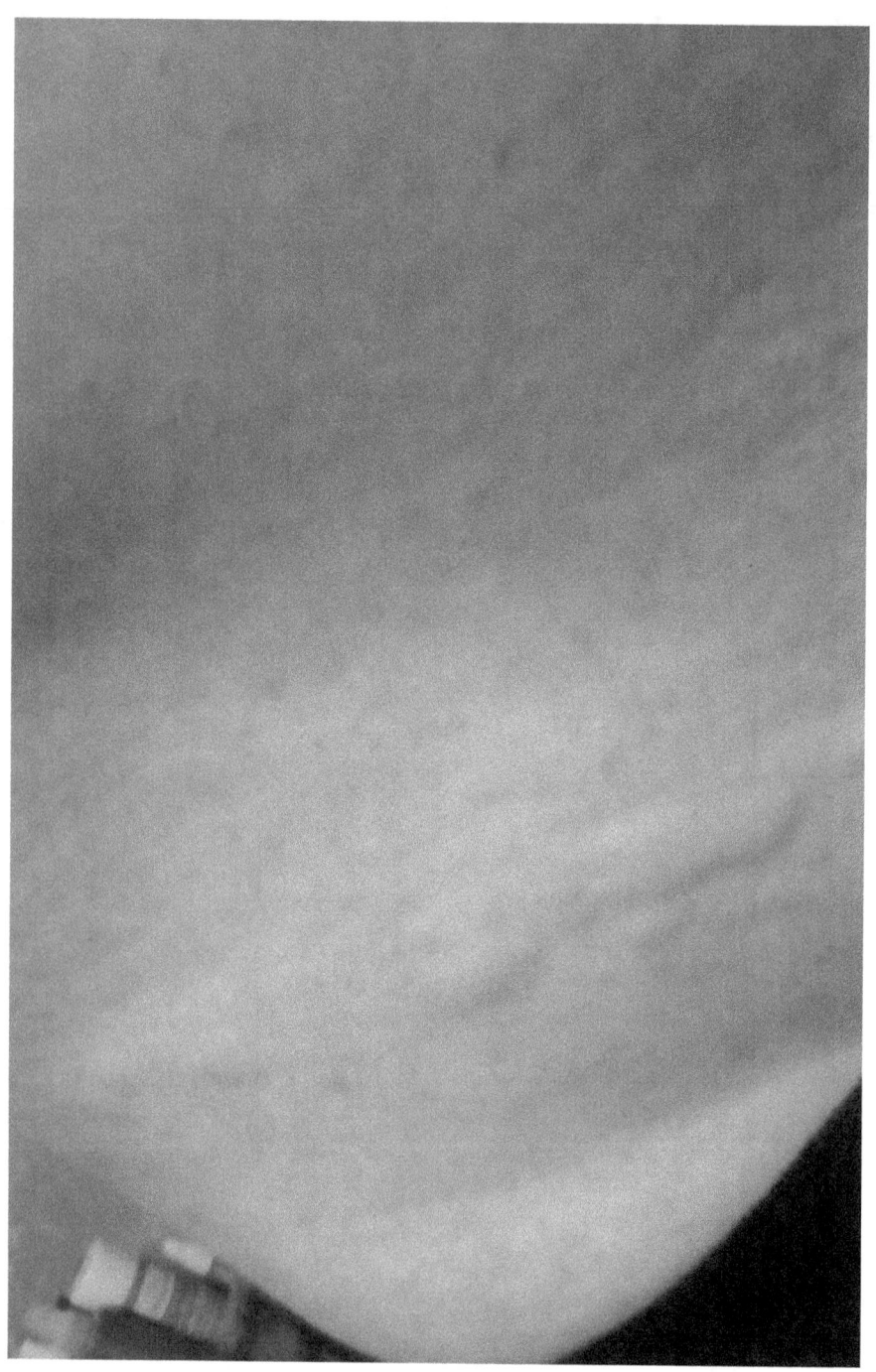

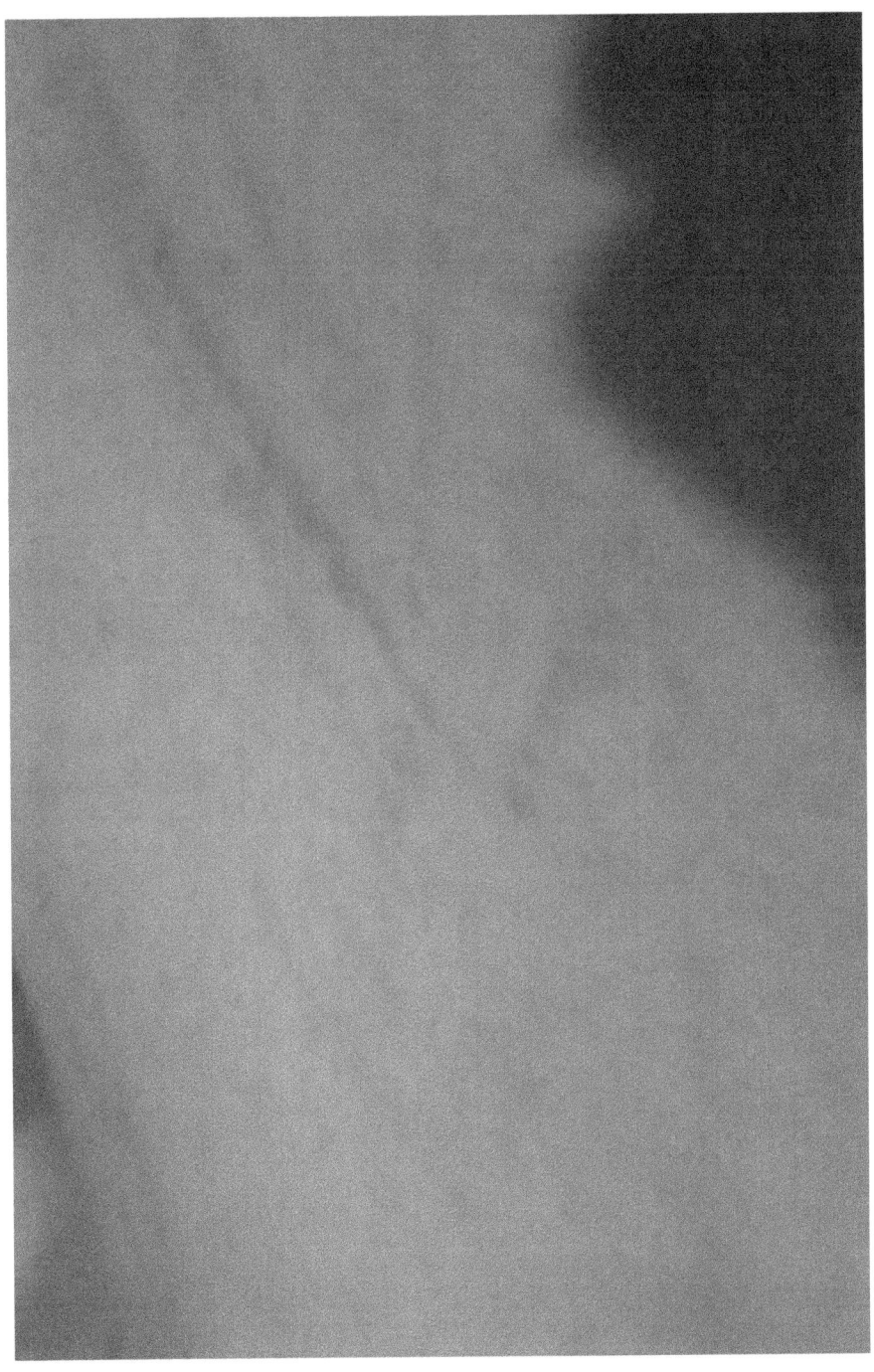

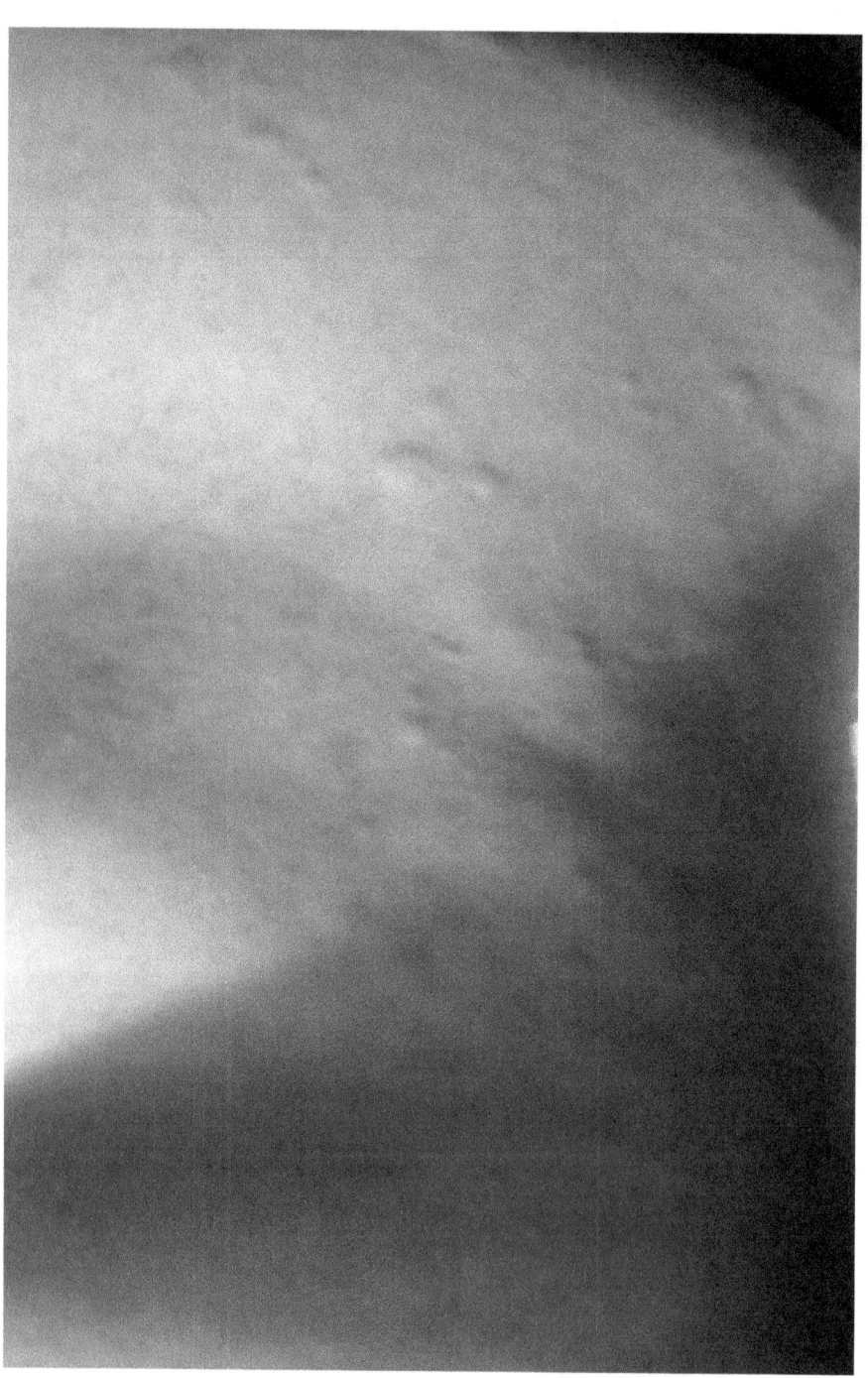

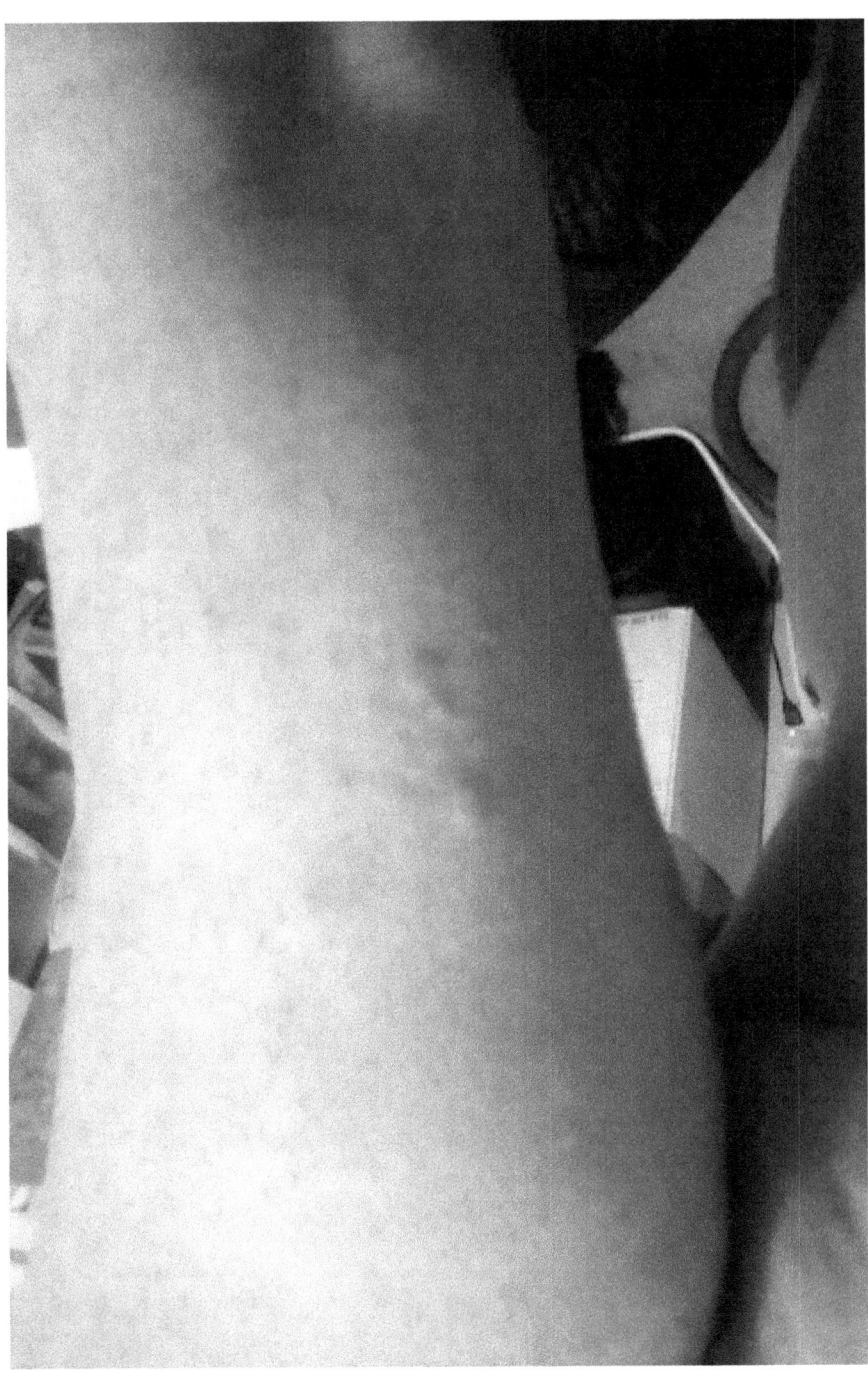

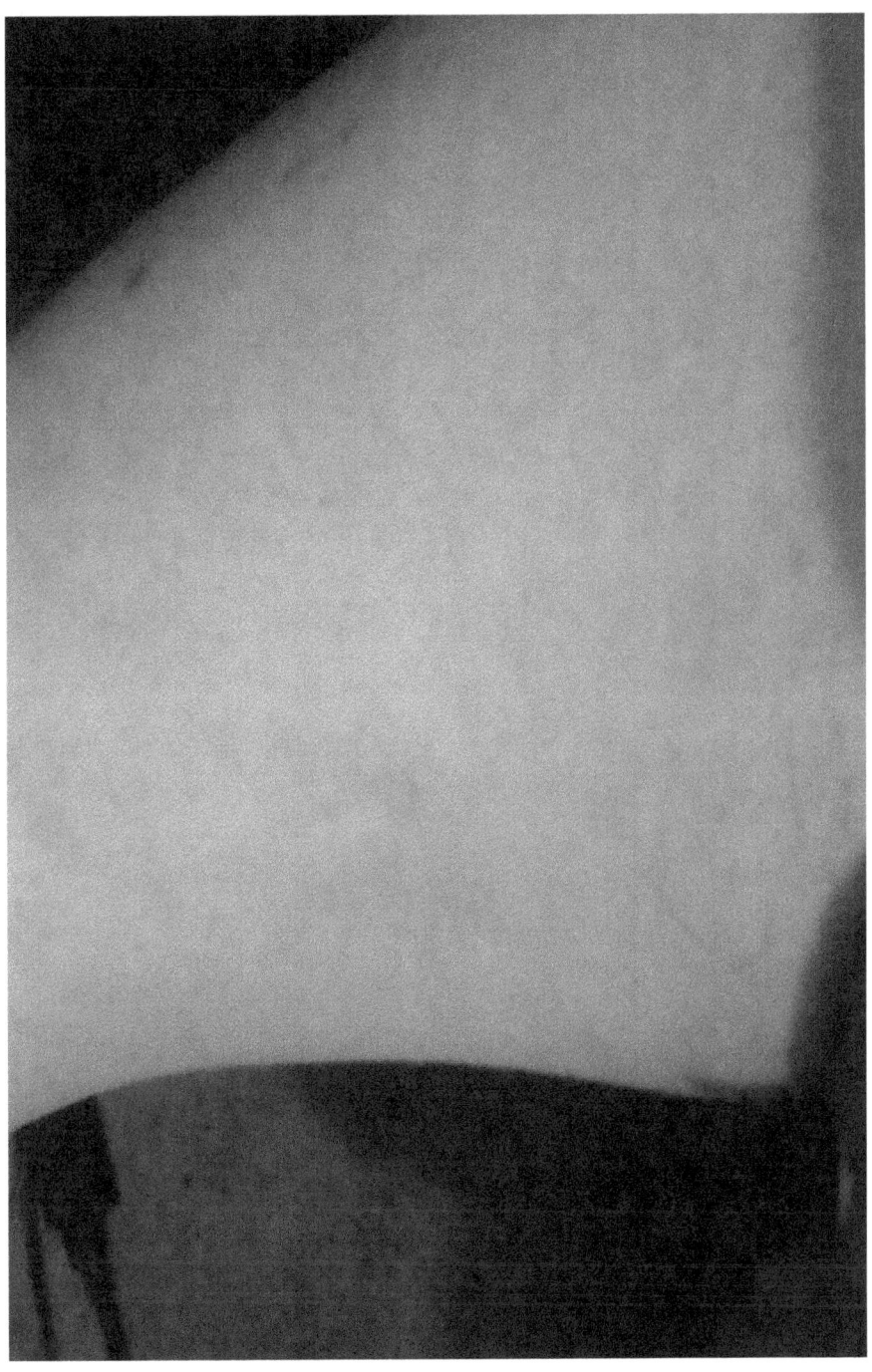

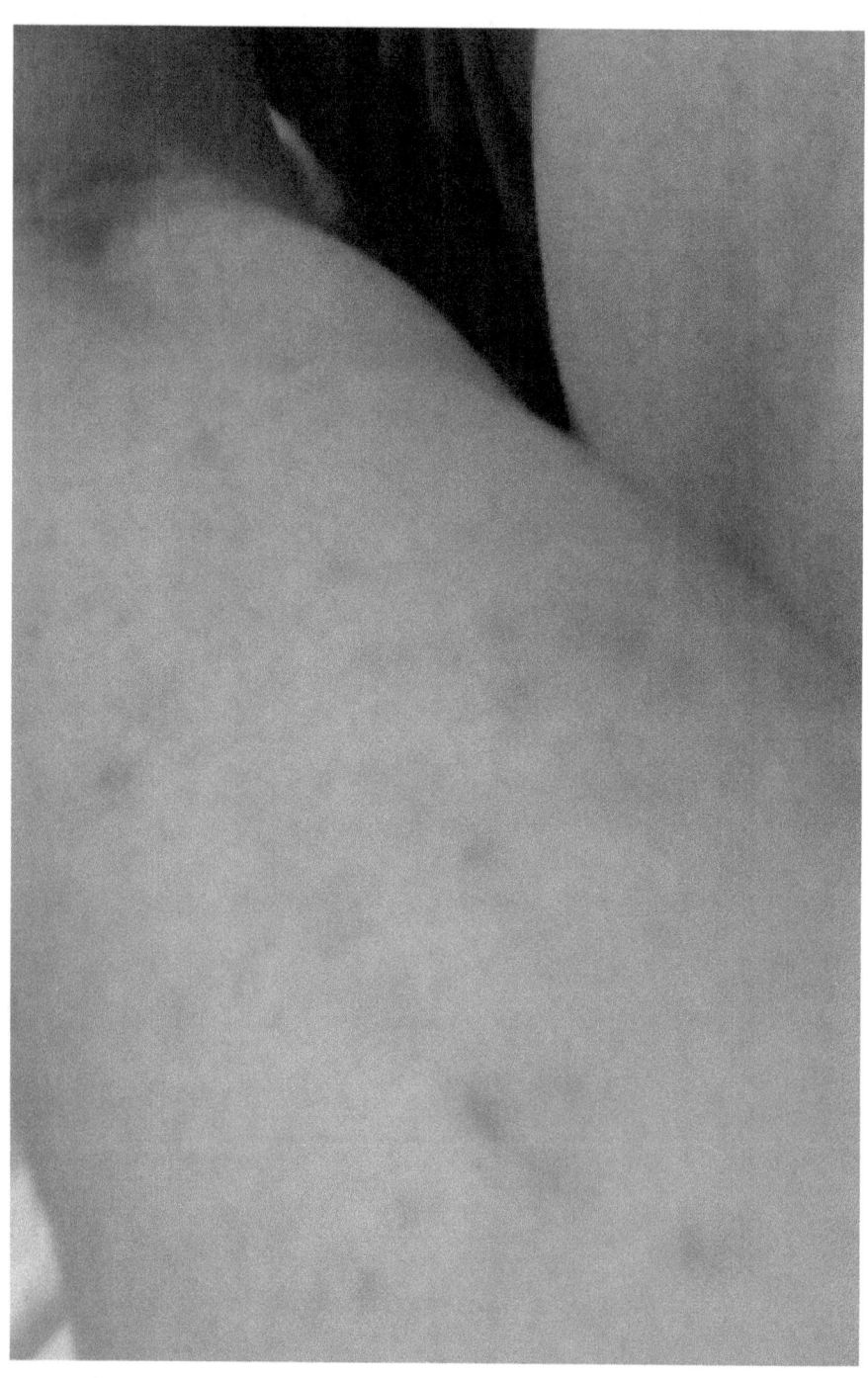

33

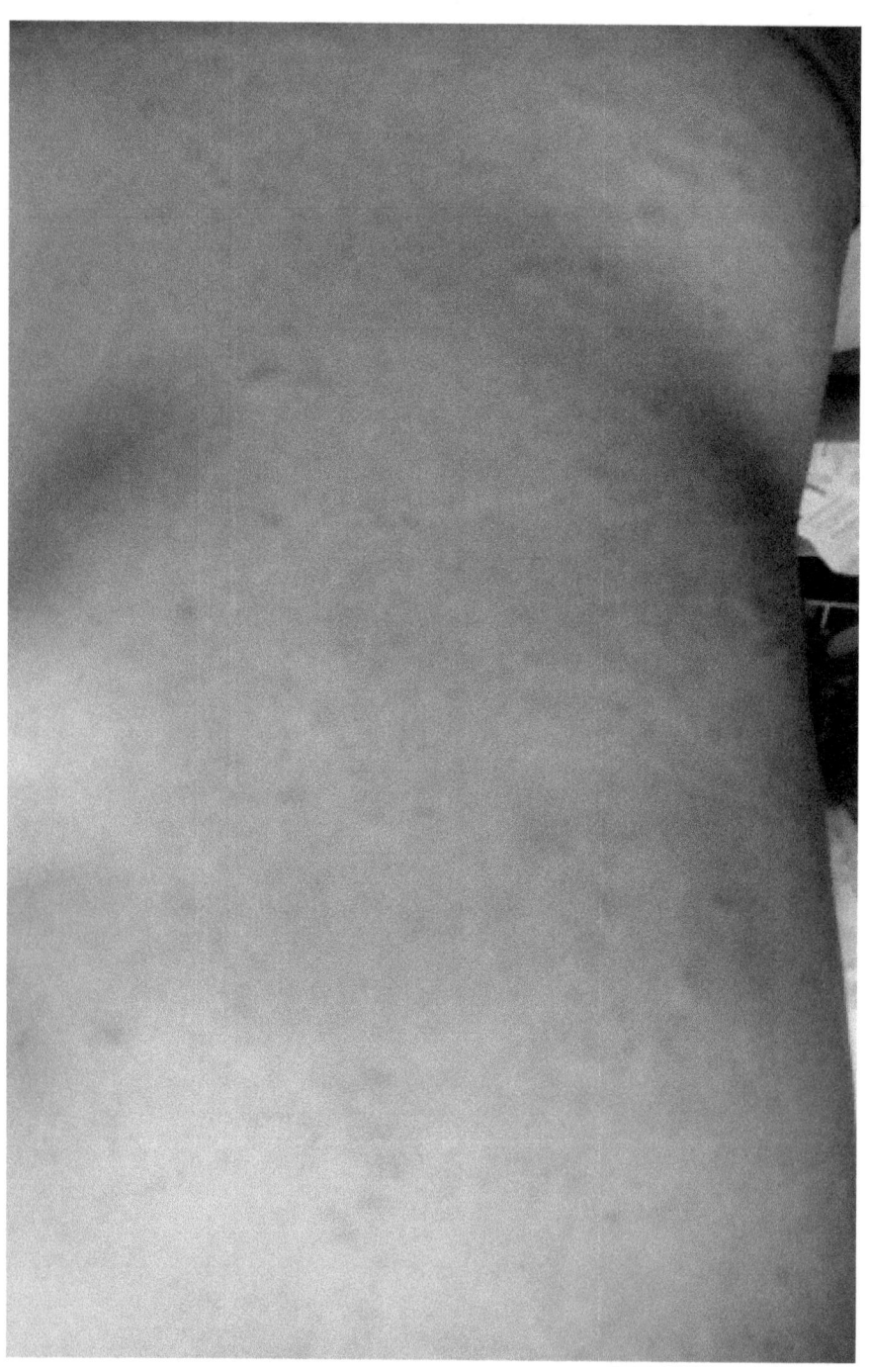

35

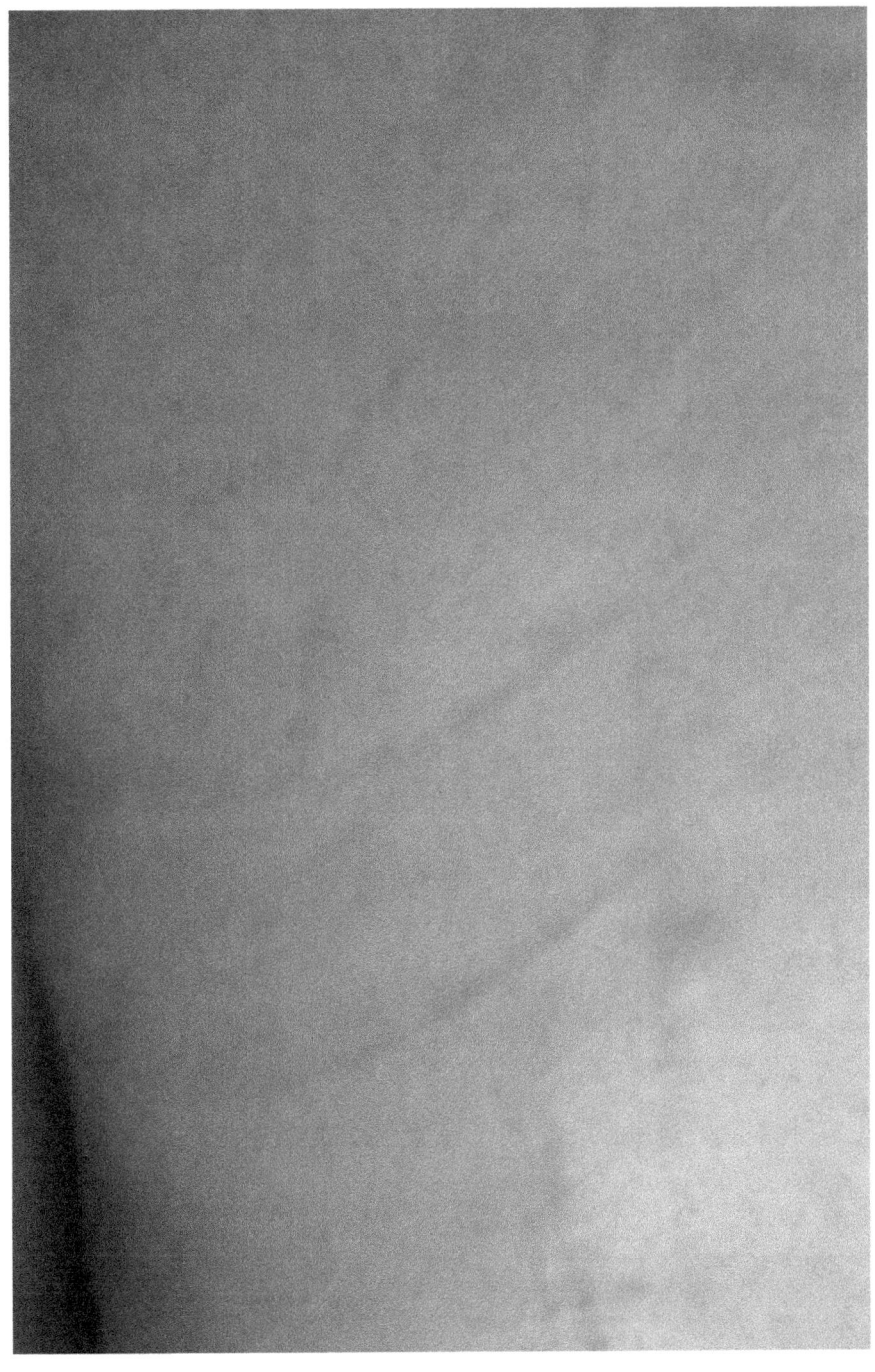

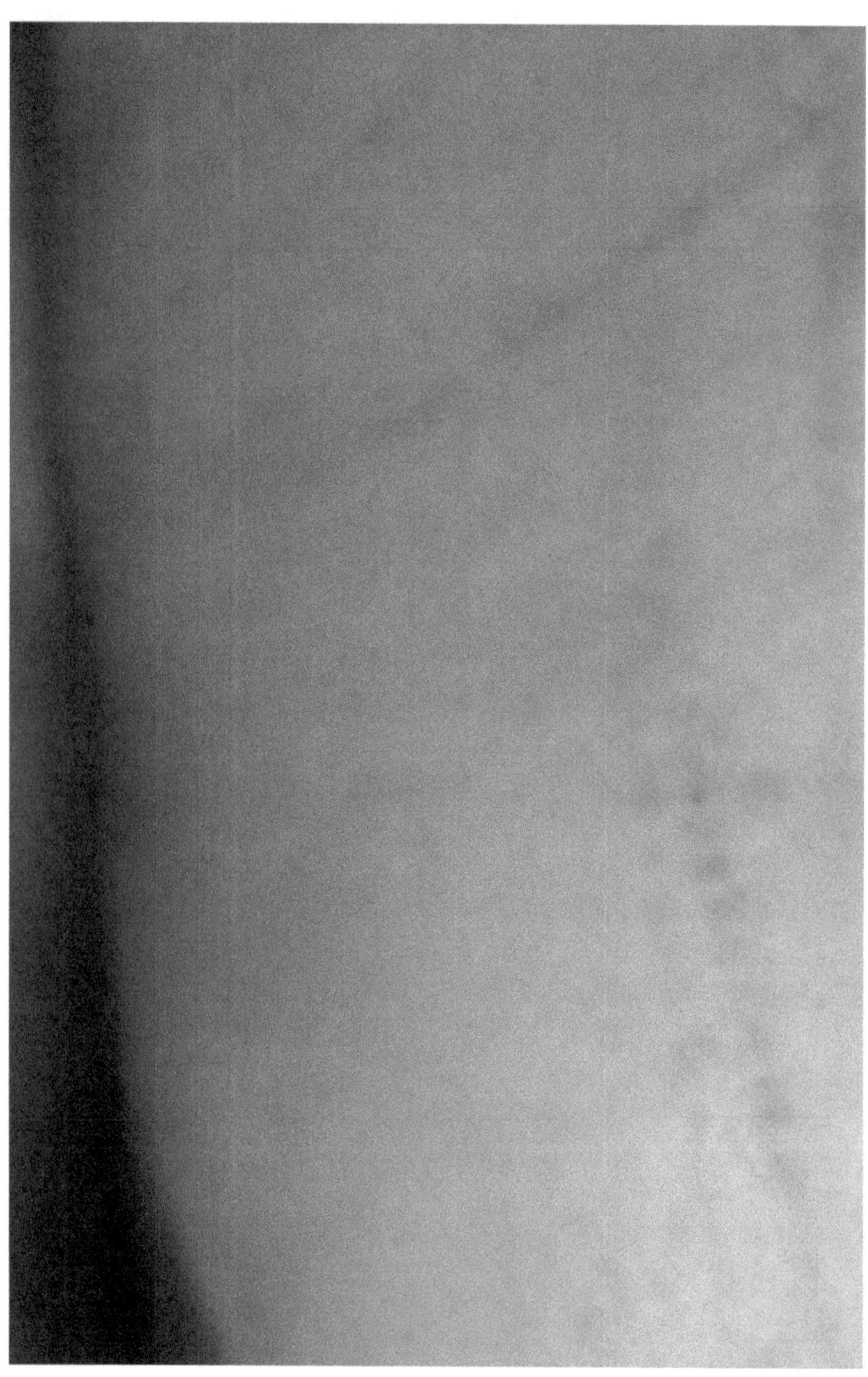

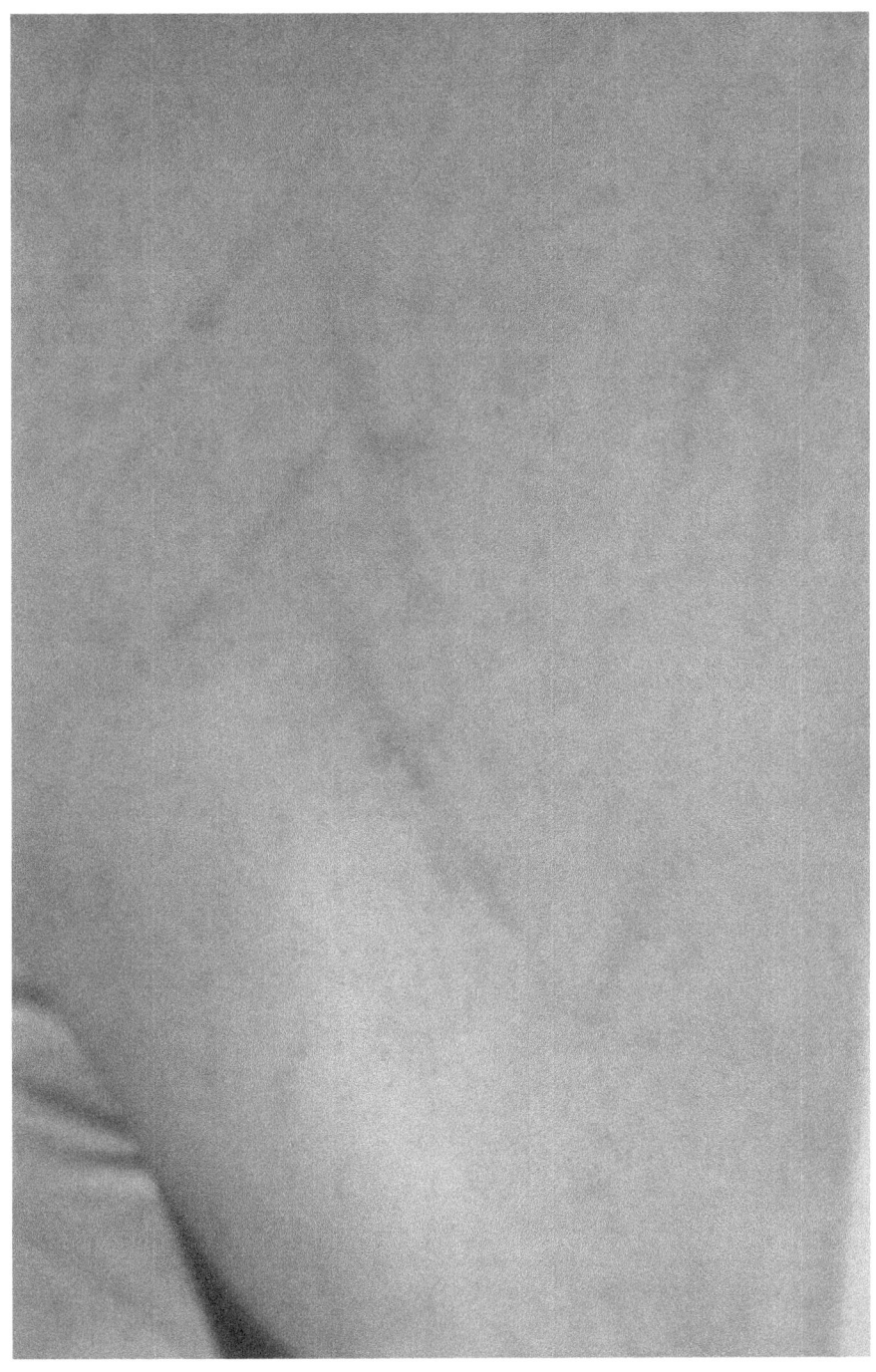

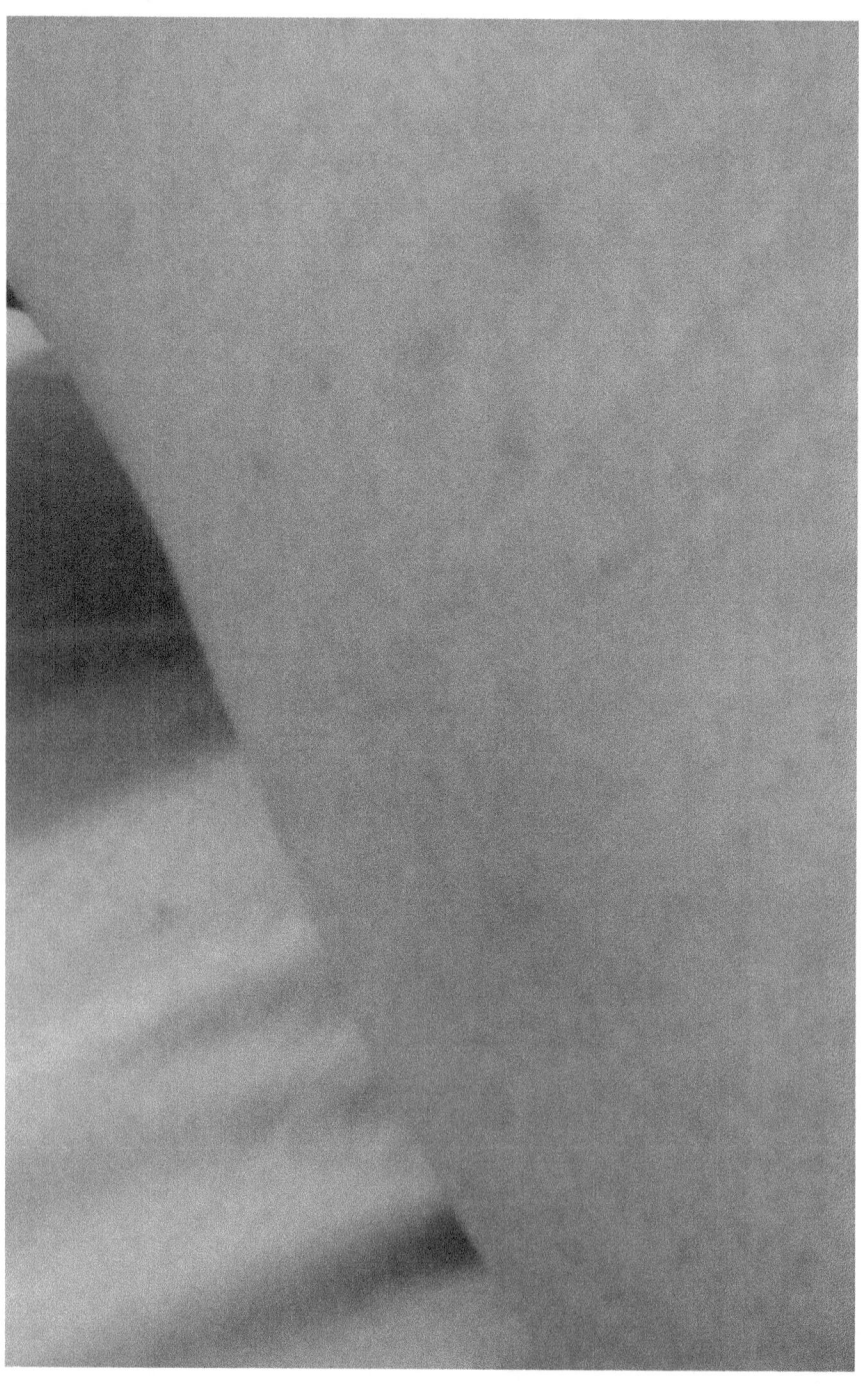

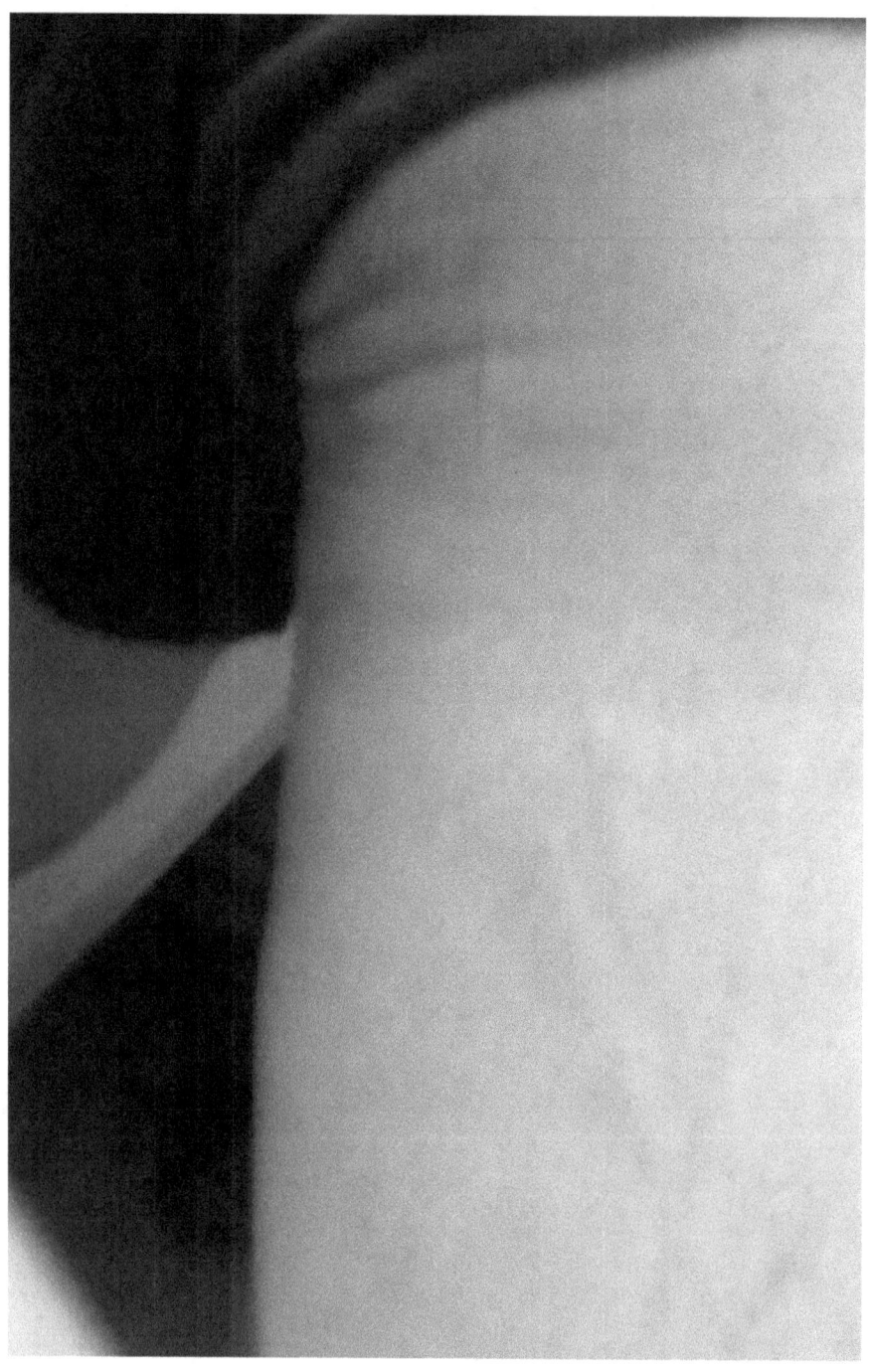

46

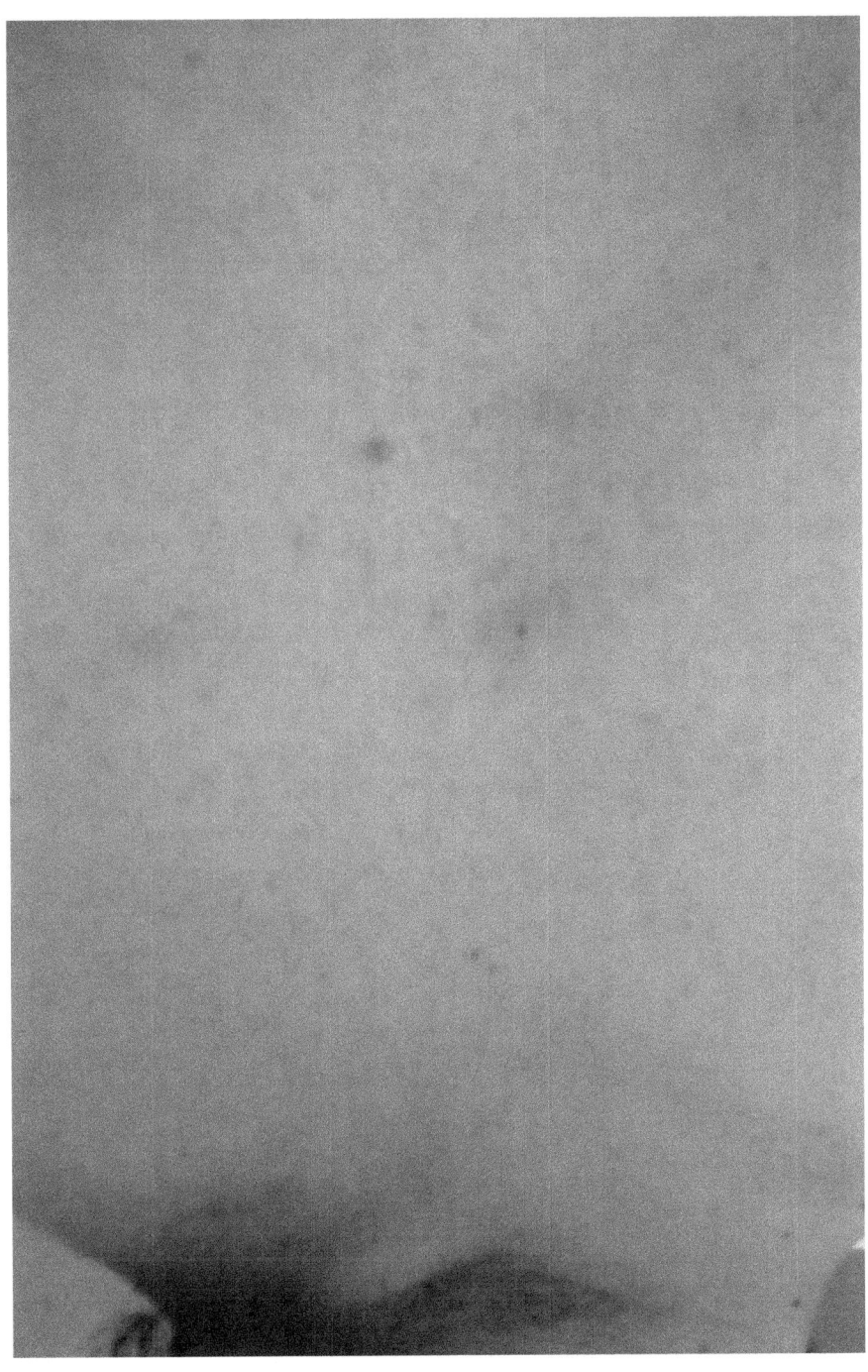

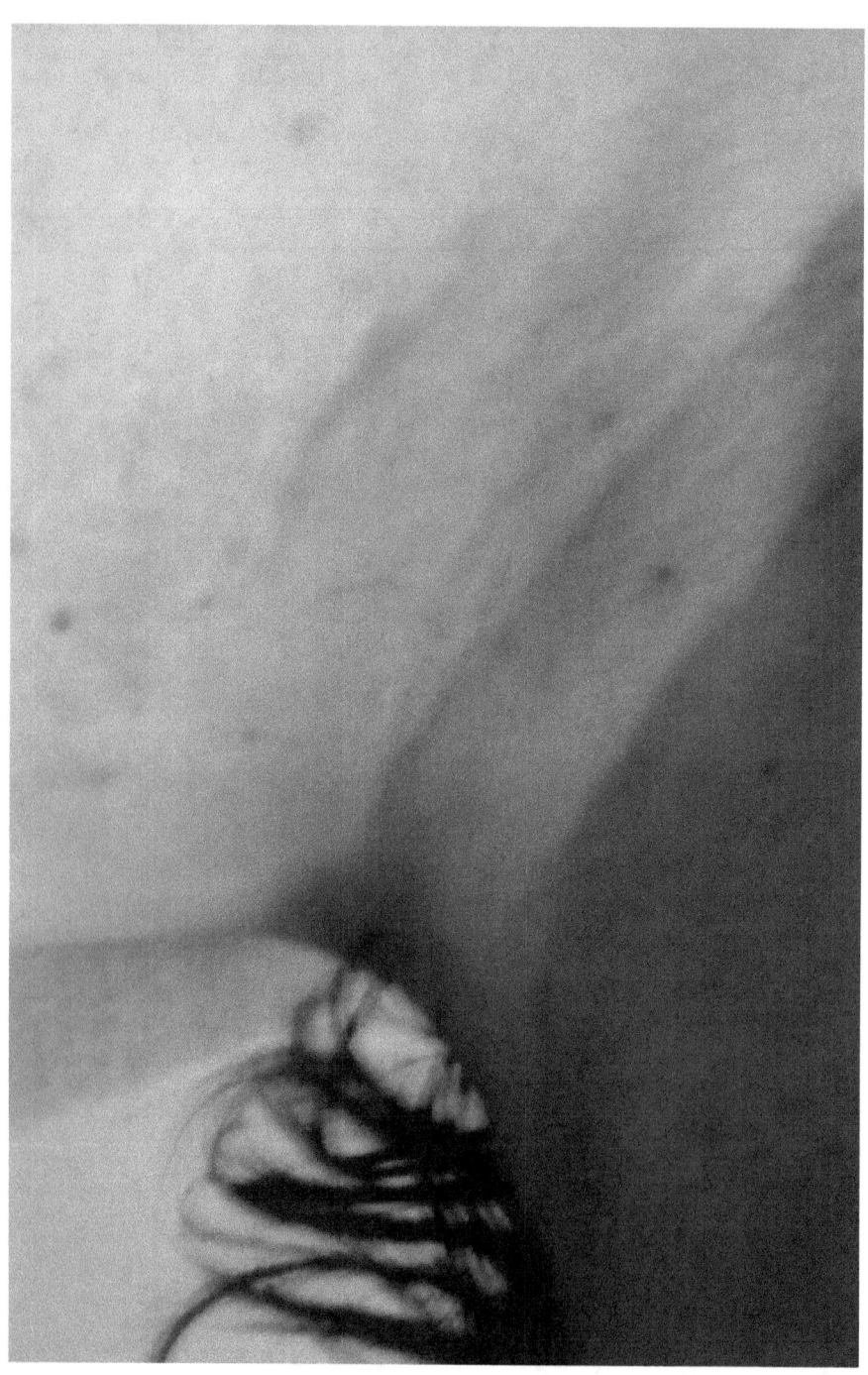

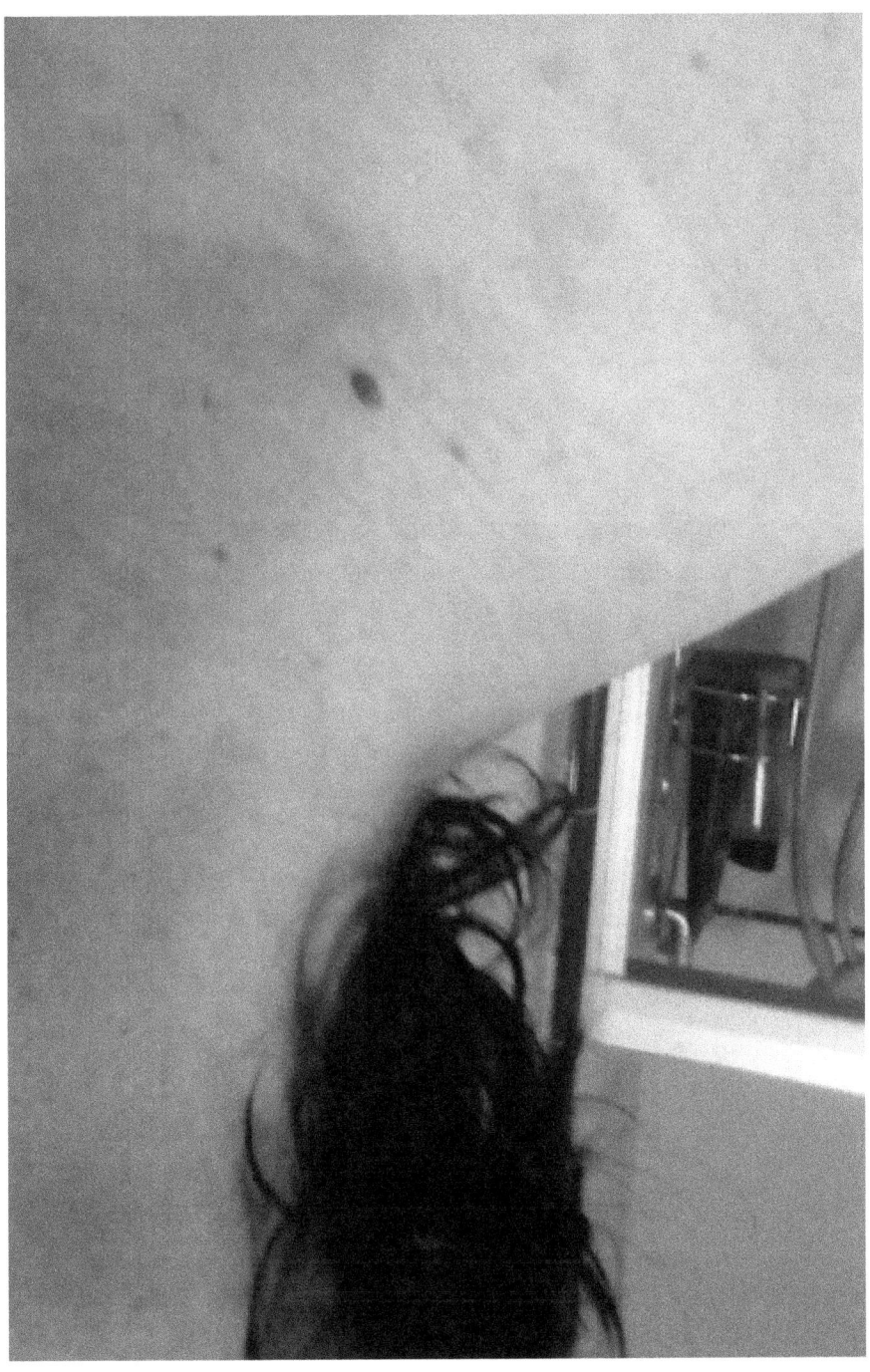

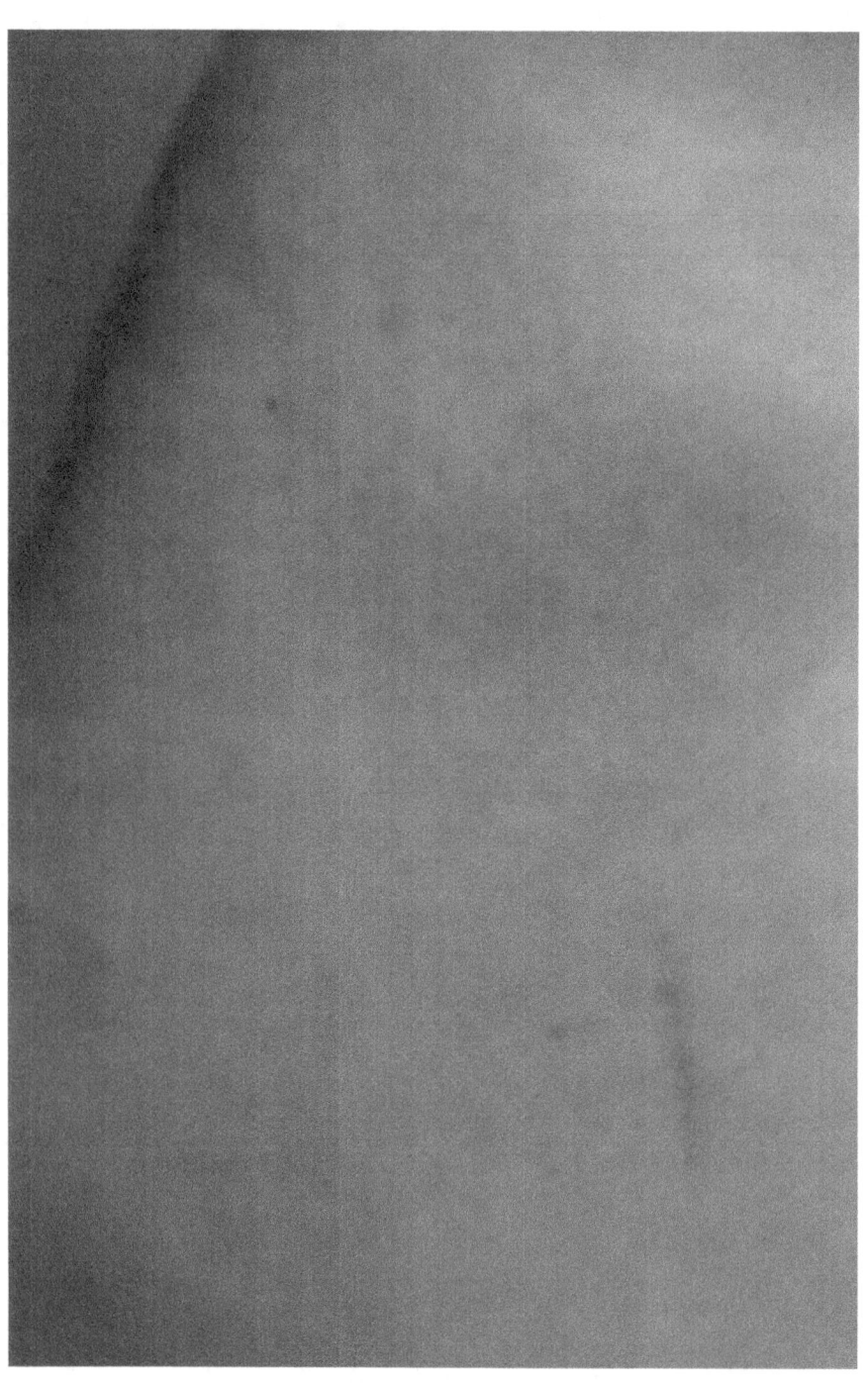

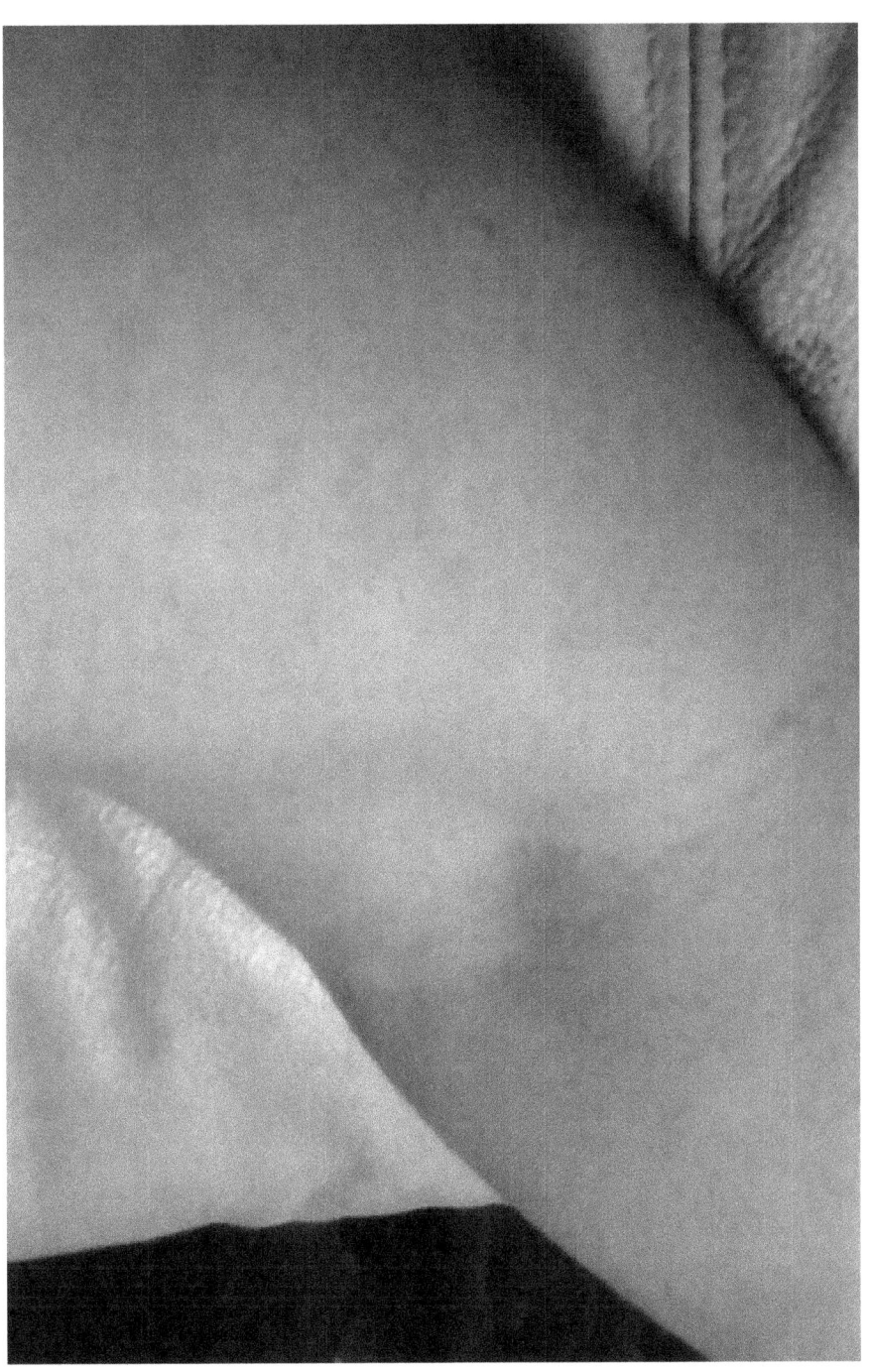

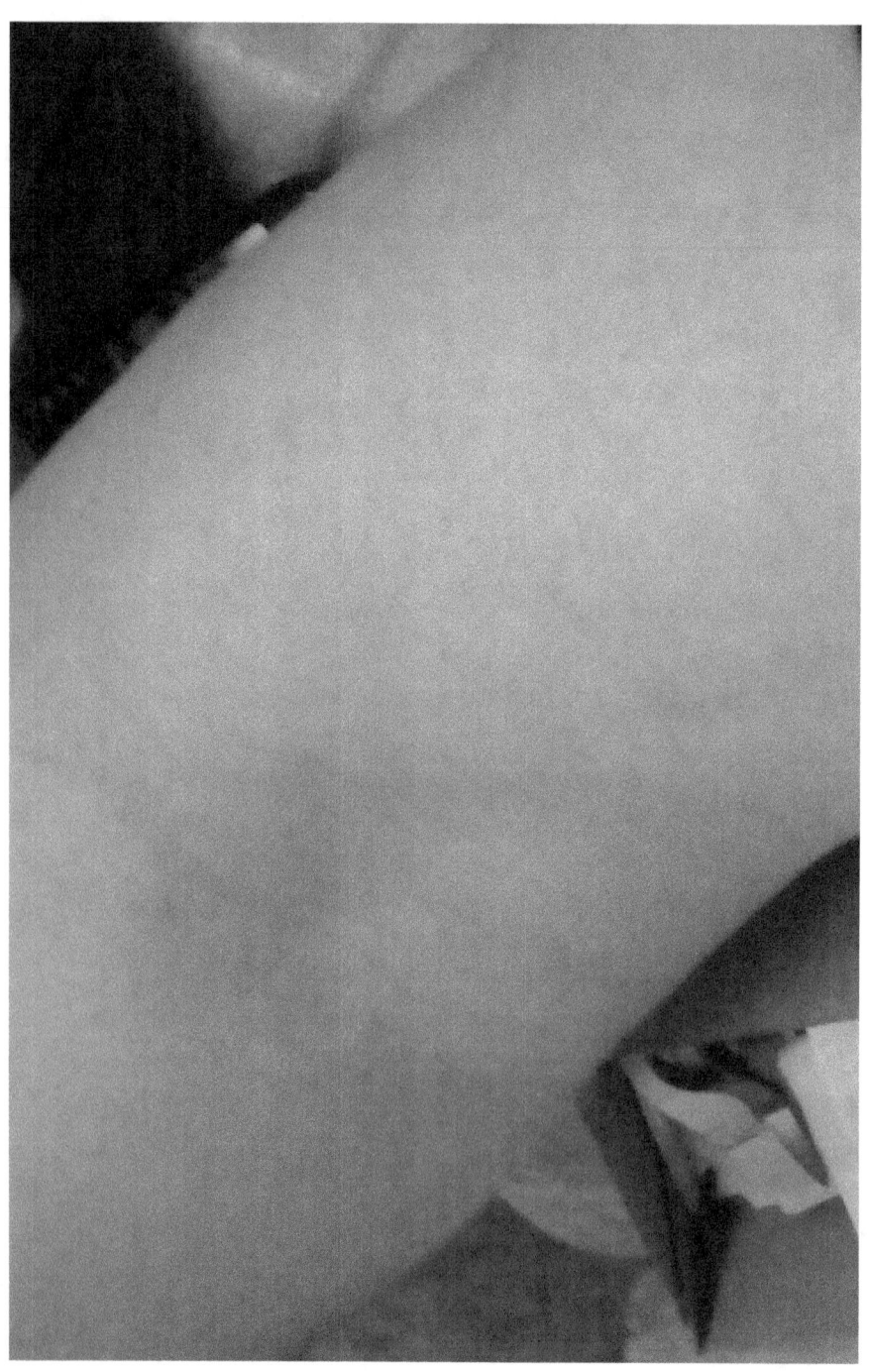

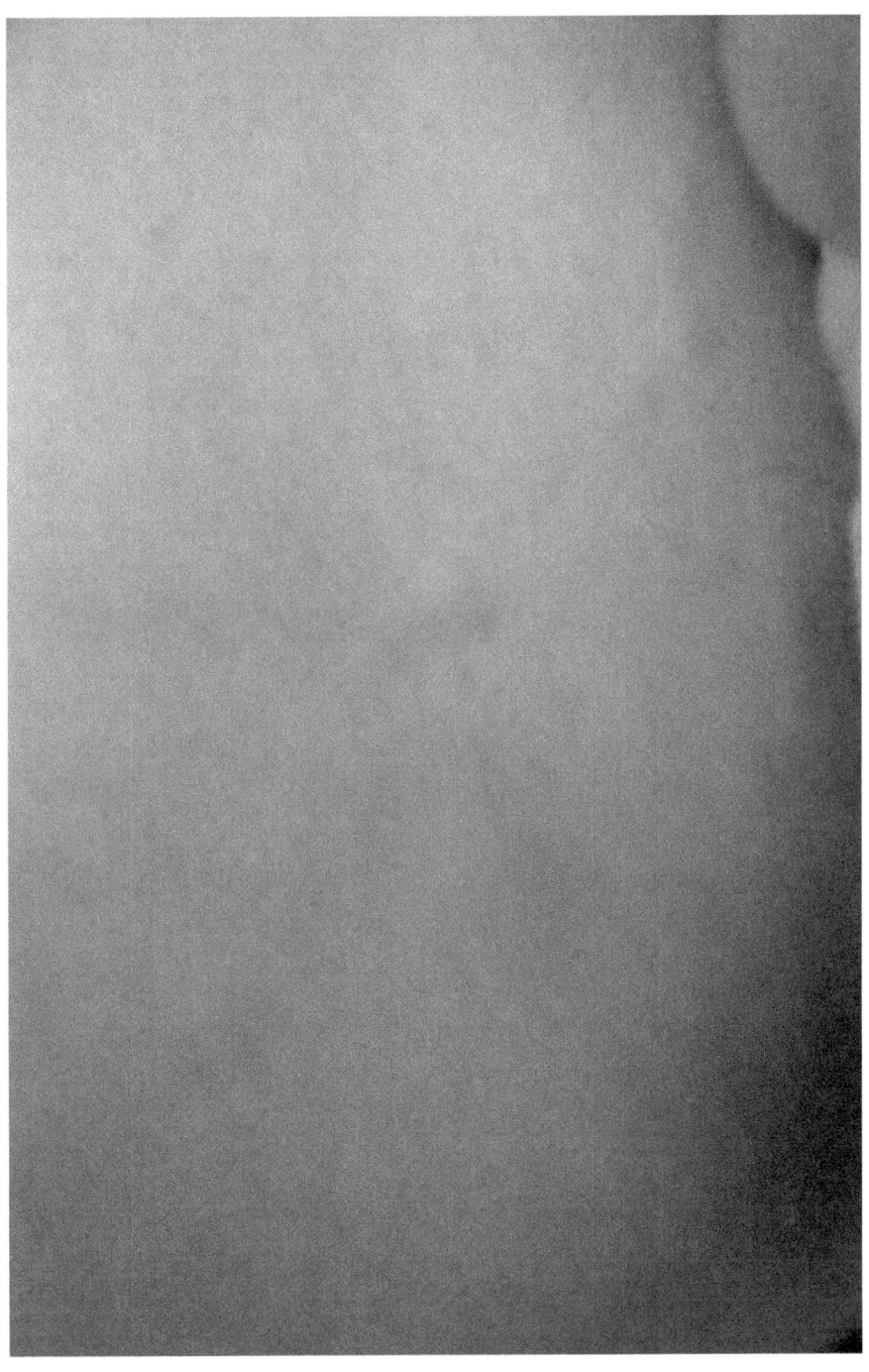

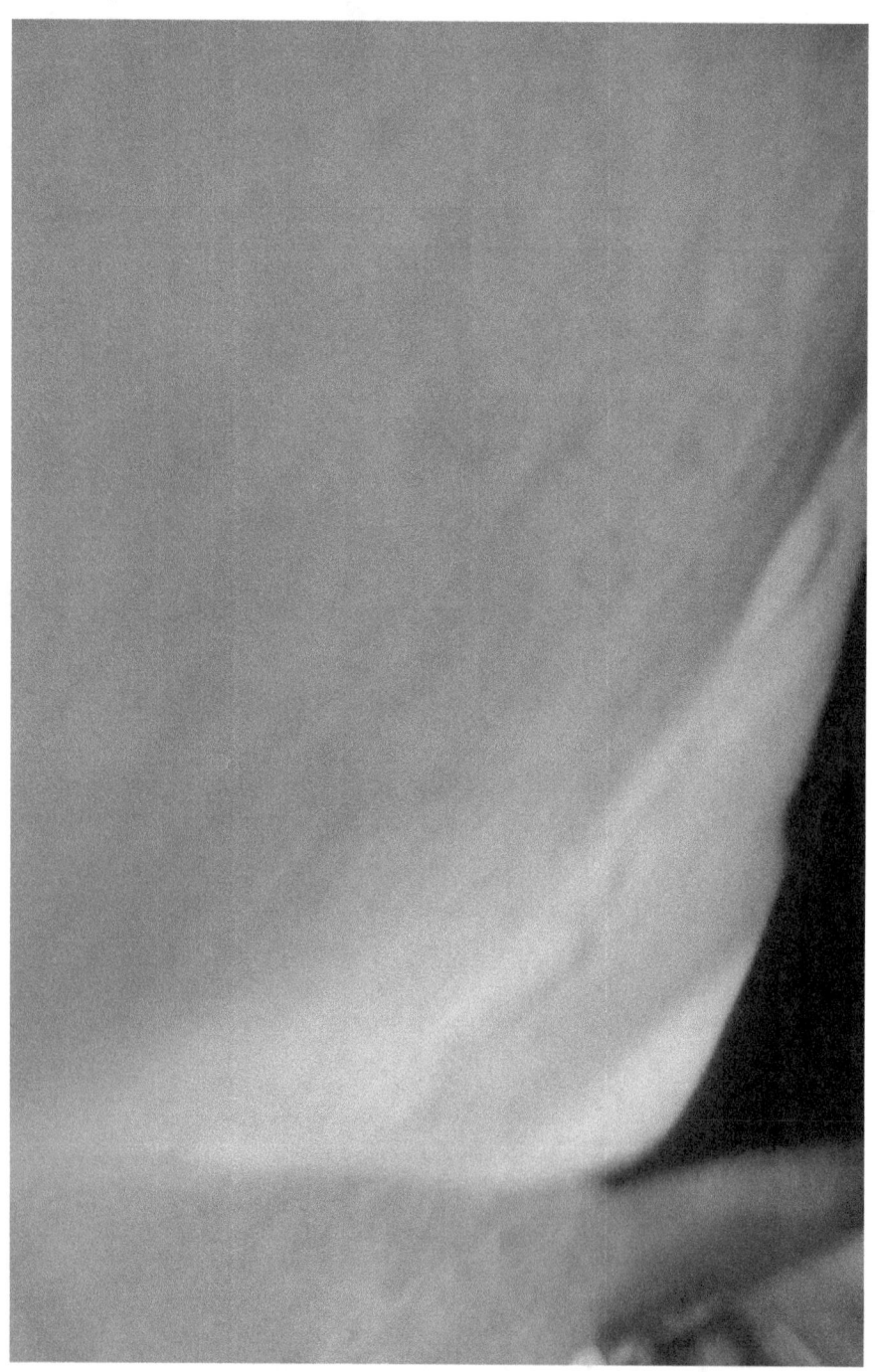

65

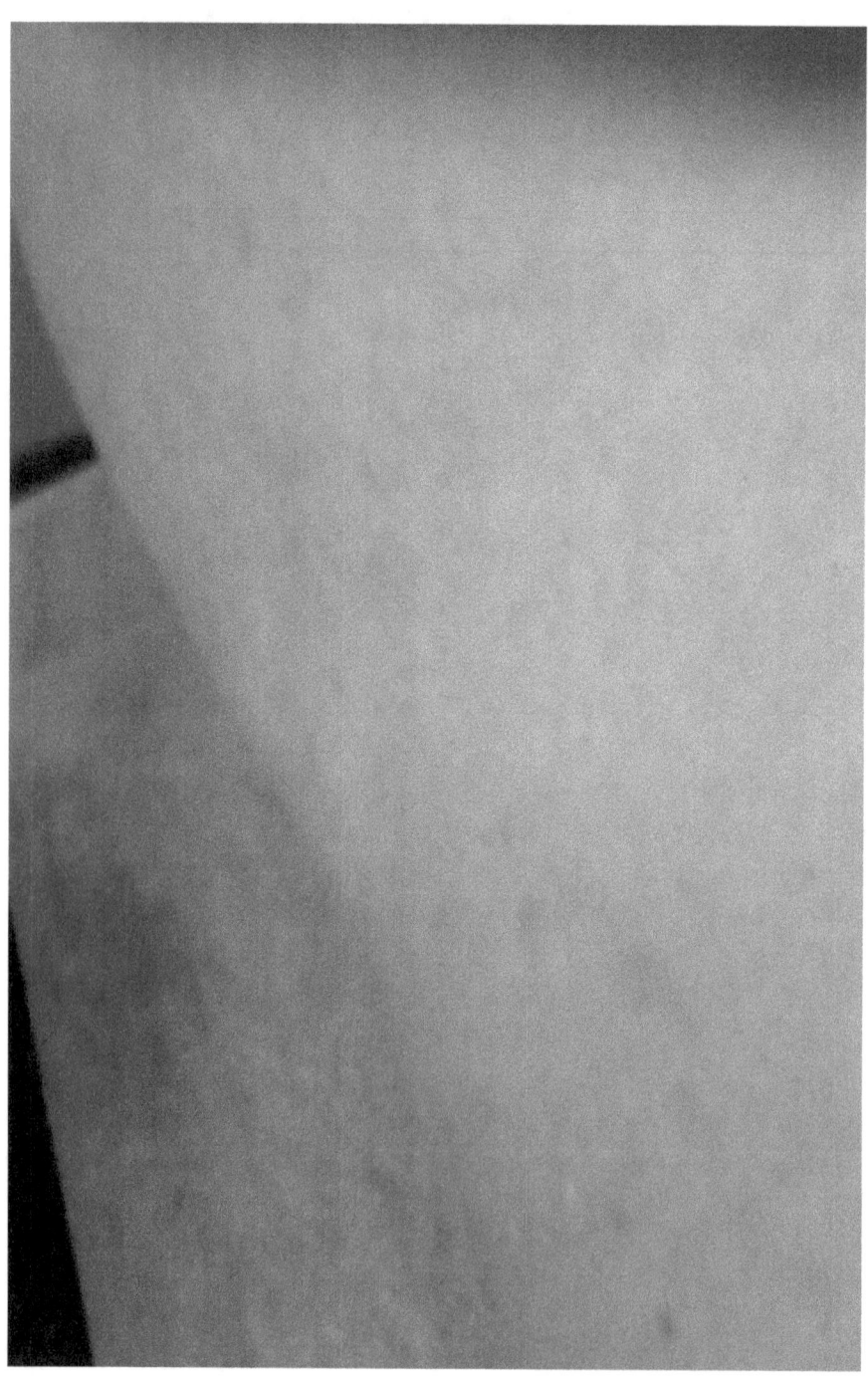

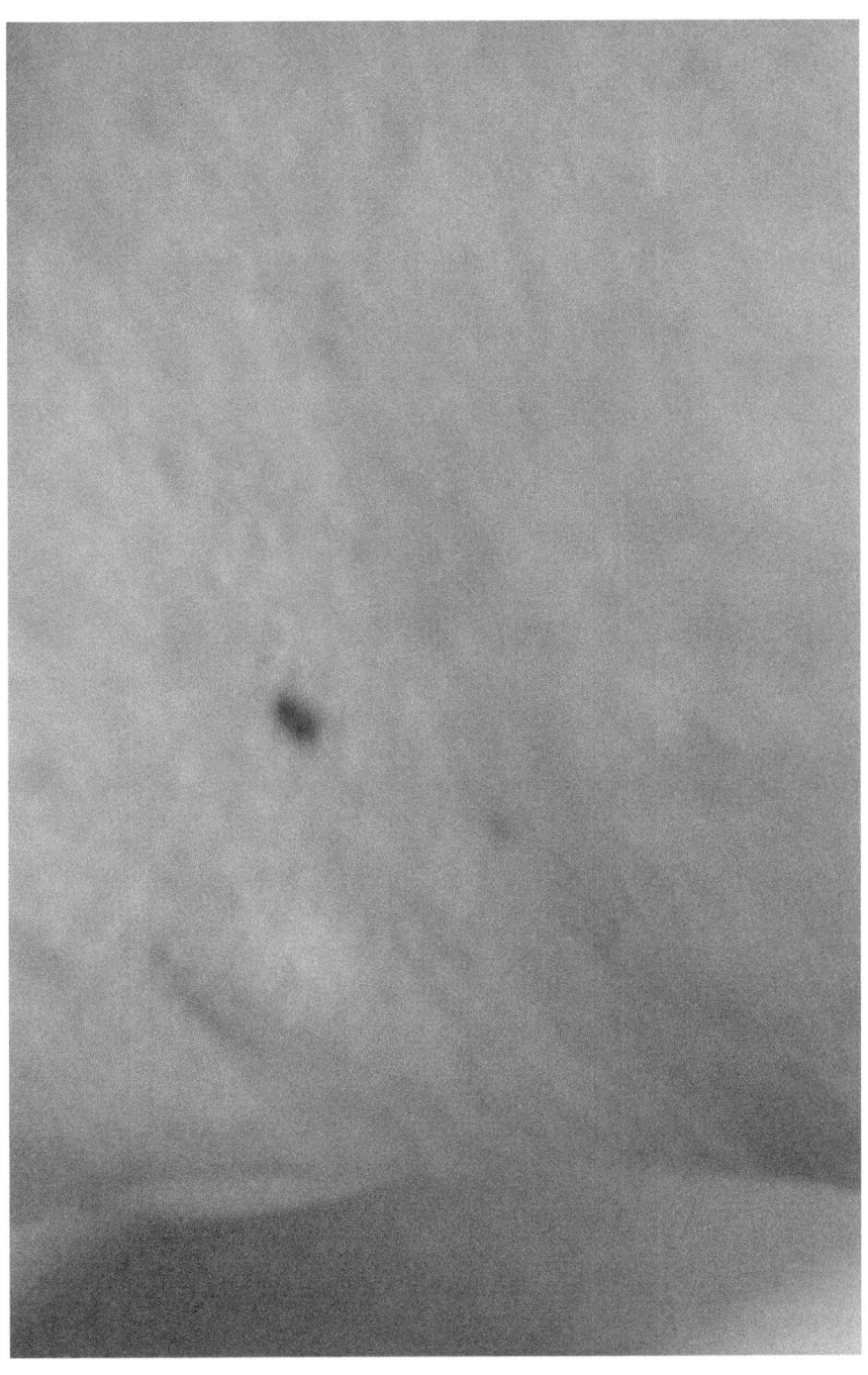

77

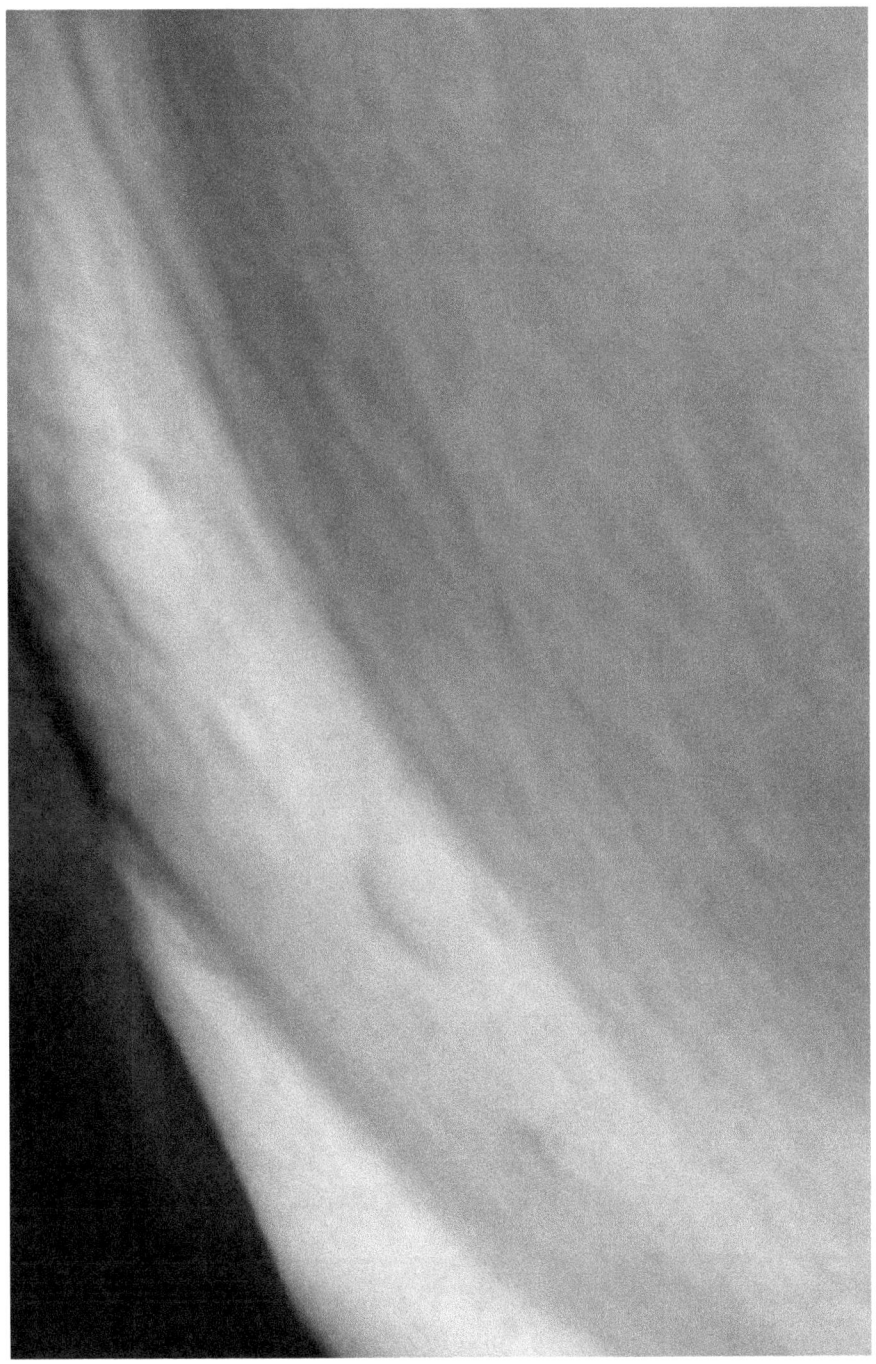

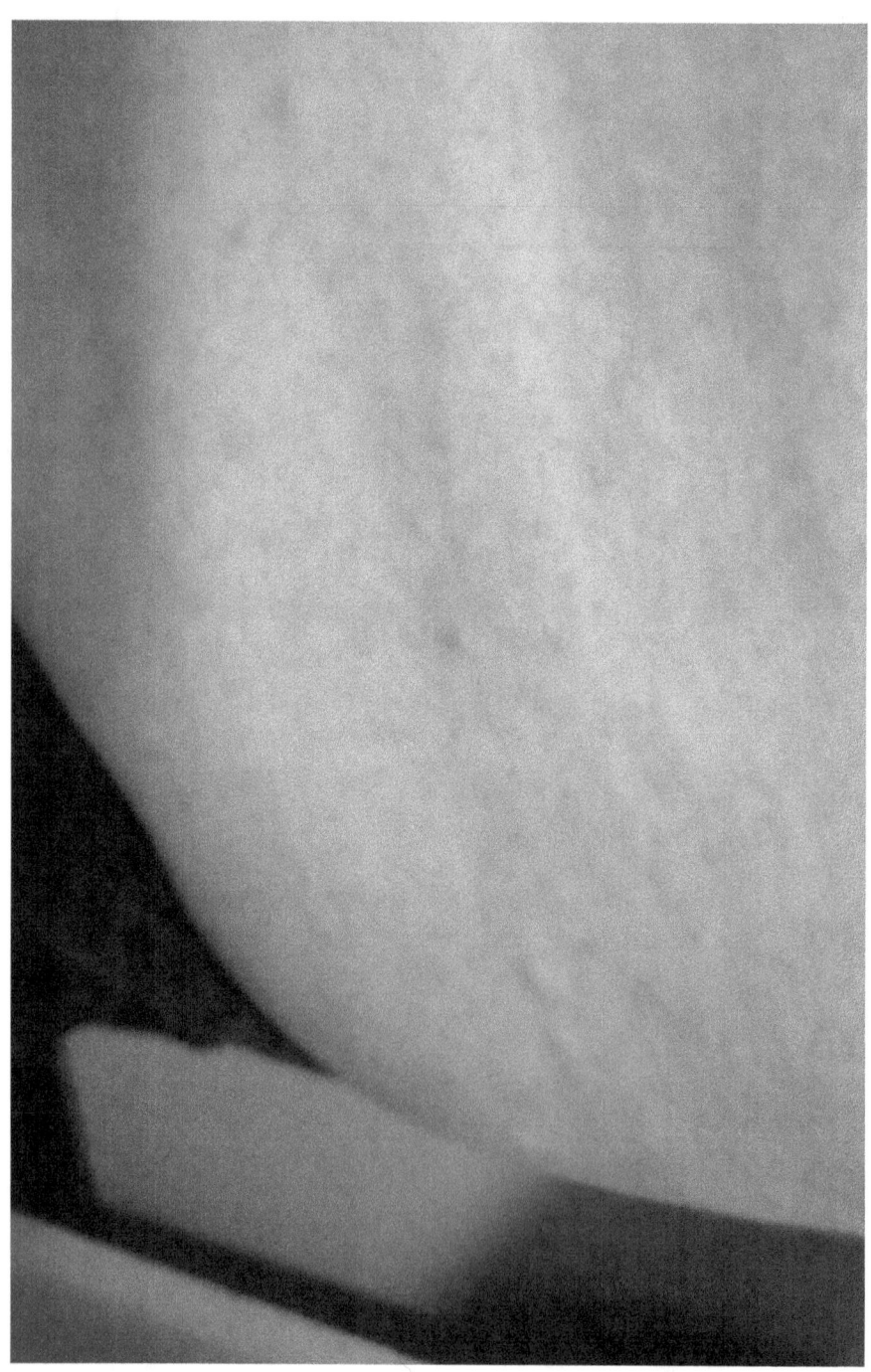

77

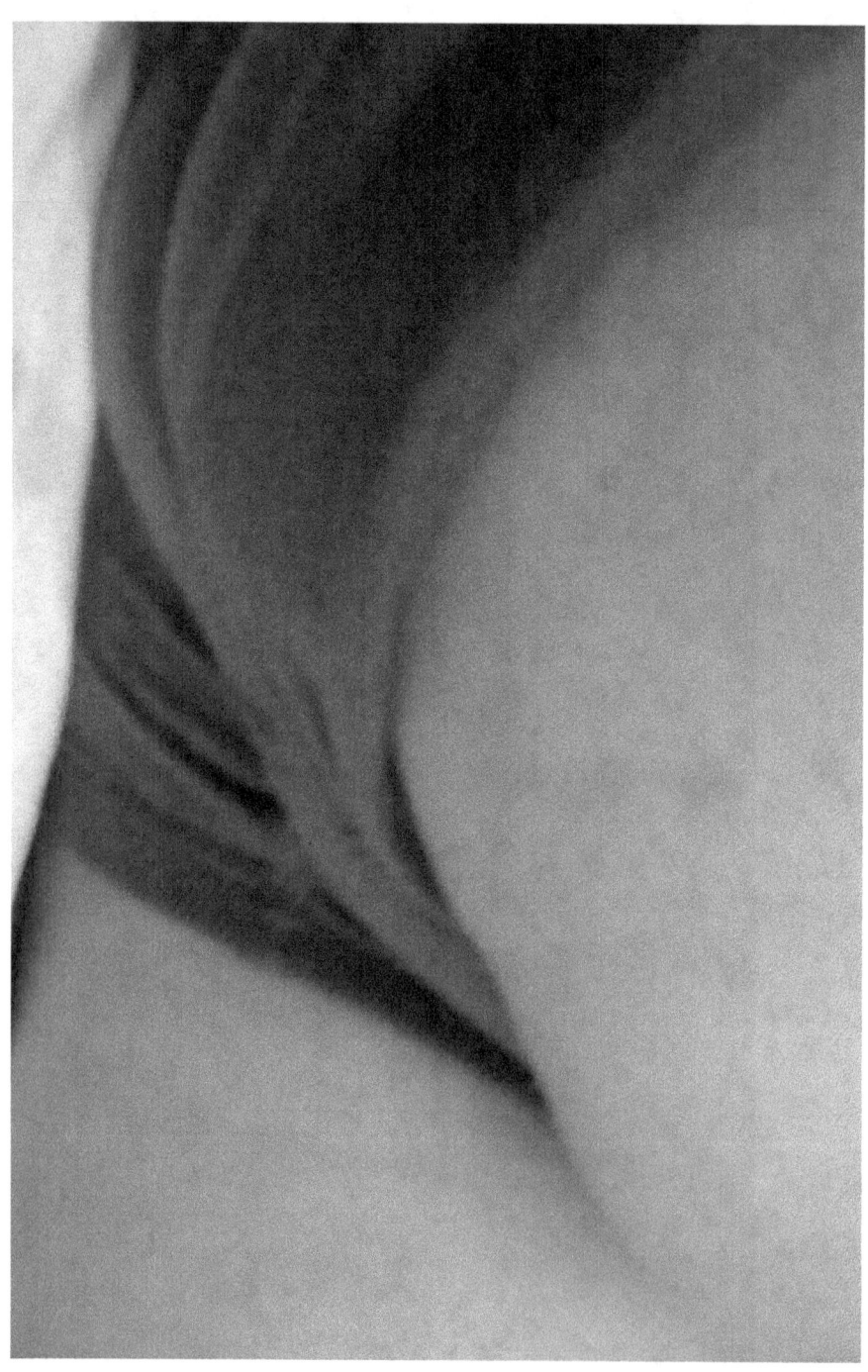

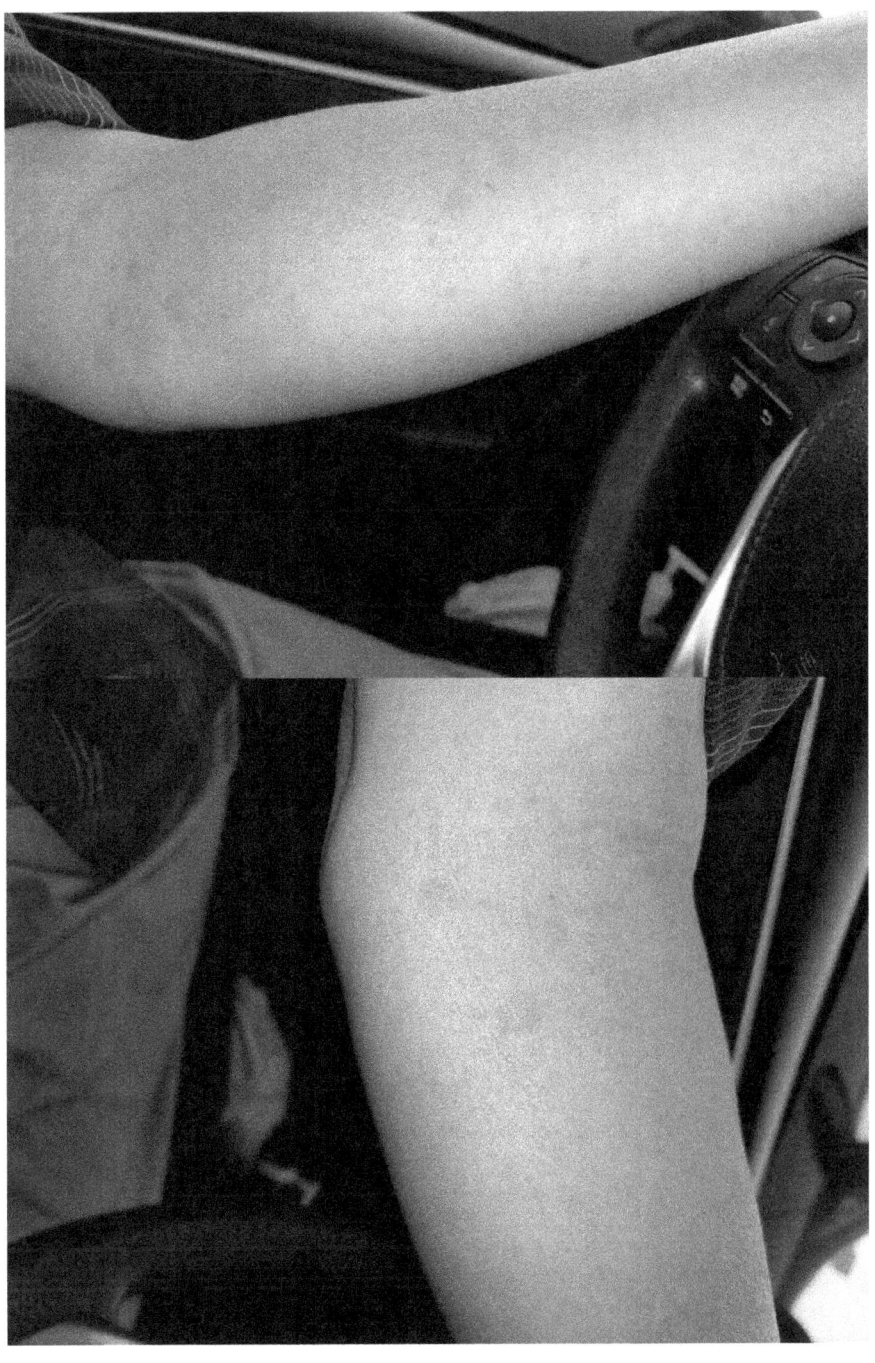

www.ingramcontent.com/pod-product-compliance
Lightning Source LLC
Chambersburg PA
CBHW052337220526

45472CB00001B/463